Fit to Practice

Rochester Studies in Medical History

Senior Editor: Theodore M. Brown
Professor of History and Preventive Medicine
University of Rochester

Additional Titles of Interest

Save the Babies: American Public Health Reform and the Prevention of Infant Mortality, 1850–1929
Richard A. Meckel

Intrusive Interventions: Public Health, Domestic Space, and Infectious Disease Surveillance in England, 1840–1914
Graham Mooney

The Antivaccine Heresy: "Jacobson v. Massachusetts" and the Troubled History of Compulsory Vaccination in the United States
Karen L. Walloch

Healthy Boundaries: Property, Law, and Public Health in England and Wales, 1815–1872
James G. Hanley

Psychiatry and Racial Liberalism in Harlem, 1936–1968
Dennis A. Doyle

Childbirth, Maternity, and Medical Pluralism in French Colonial Vietnam, 1880–1945
Thuy Linh Nguyen

Setting Nutritional Standards: Theory, Policies, Practices
Edited by Elizabeth Neswald, David F. Smith, and Ulrike Thoms

Technological Change in Modern Surgery: Historical Perspectives on Innovation
Edited by Thomas Schlich and Christopher Crenner

The History of the Brain and Mind Sciences: Technique, Technology, Therapy
Edited by Stephen T. Casper and Delia Gavrus

Reasoning against Madness: Psychiatry and the State in Rio de Janeiro, 1830–1944
Manuella Meyer

A complete list of titles in the Rochester Studies in Medical History series may be found on our website, www.urpress.com.

Fit to Practice

Empire, Race, Gender, and the Making of British Medicine, 1850–1980

Douglas M. Haynes

University of Rochester Press

First published 2017

University of Rochester Press
668 Mt. Hope Avenue, Rochester, NY 14620, USA
www.urpress.com
and Boydell & Brewer Limited
PO Box 9, Woodbridge, Suffolk IP12 3DF, UK
www.boydellandbrewer.com

ISBN-13: 978-1-58046-581-6
ISSN: 1526-2715

Library of Congress Cataloging-in-Publication Data

Names: Haynes, Douglas Melvin, author.
Title: Fit to practice : empire, race, gender, and the making of British medicine, 1850–1980 / Douglas M. Haynes.
Description: Rochester, NY : University of Rochester Press, 2017. | Series: Rochester studies in medical history, ISSN 1526-2715 ; vol. 42 | Includes bibliographical references and index.
Identifiers: LCCN 2017031776 | ISBN 9781580465816 (hardcover : alk. paper)
Subjects: LCSH: Medicine—Great Britain—History—19th century. | Medicine—Great Britain—History—20th century. | Discrimination in medical care—Great Britain. | Medical policy—Social aspects—Great Britain.
Classification: LCC R486 .H39 2017 | DDC 610.941—dc23 LC record available at https://lccn.loc.gov/2017031776

A catalogue record for this title is available from the British Library.

This publication is printed on acid-free paper.
Printed in the United States of America.

Contents

Acknowledgments

Authorship is at once a solitary enterprise and a product of an intellectual community. I have been very fortunate in having a supportive and generous community of colleagues, librarians, archivists, and editors. I want to thank my history colleagues at the University of California at Irvine for their encouragement from the conception to completion of this book as well as the Humanities Commons for a grant in support of the publication of the manuscript. Throughout this process, archivists at the National Archives (Kew), Royal College of Physicians, Royal College of Surgeons of England, Wellcome Institute, and Worshipful Society Apothecaries, one and all, guided me to valuable sources that yielded scholarly communications. Even before the book began to take shape, I benefited from the insights and engagement of scholars at various seminars, conferences, and research meetings in Britain and the United States. The sponsoring organizations include Green College, Oxford University; the University of Kansas Medical Center; and Huntington Library in San Marino, California. Several early publications appeared in collections edited by David Arnold, Philippa Levine and Kevin Grant, and Dane Kennedy and Durba Ghosh. Their careful reading and constructive criticism contributed to the momentum of the larger project. One of the pleasures of writing the manuscript was the partnership that I enjoyed with my doctoral student, Cherish Bolton, who provided inspired research assistance. The team at the University of Rochester Press as well as the reviewers was invaluable in providing thoughtful direction for revising the manuscript for publication. I especially want to thank Ted Brown, editor of the Rochester Studies in Medical History, for his sage advice and the professionalism of assistant editor Julia Cook. Finally, I want to thank my wife, Cherie, for being a wonderful partner throughout this intellectual odyssey and my son, Zachary, and my daughter, Alaina, for being a profound source of pride.

Abbreviations

BMA	British Medical Association
CAB	Cabinet Office
GMC	General Medical Council
ECFMG	US Educational Council Foreign Medical Graduate Examination
EEC	European Economic Community
IMS	Indian Medical Service
JCC	Joint Consultants Committee
MH	Ministry of Health
NHS	National Health Service
PC	Privy Council, or Privy Office
PLAB	Professional Linguistic Assessment Board Examination

Introduction

Since the 1950s, the presence of overseas-trained doctors of color in the National Health Service in the United Kingdom has attracted persistent attention. Their numbers, countries of origin, training and credentials, right to practice medicine, and cultural competency have all been featured in the medical and lay press. This attention to overseas doctors, a designation that includes doctors from within and outside of the British Commonwealth or former empire, certainly reflects the unprecedented pace of the globalization of the medical profession since World War II, not to mention the rise of a multiracial, multiethnic postwar society. The meaning of the term *overseas doctors* is not limited to merely describing visible changes in the diversity of the profession. It also extends to affirming presumed certainties about the identity of British medicine. The undifferentiated description of national origins as "overseas" obscures the historical connection between British medicine and its former empire in South Asia. In highlighting heterogeneity, the term also implicitly renders the domestic profession as a homogenous social unit, bounded by the distinctive experience of the British Isles. In other words, collapsing the place of origin into a single modifier "overseas" reinforces the assumption that membership in the community of British medicine is determined by birth and training in the United Kingdom while masking the influence of the wider world in the making of British medicine.

In this book I examine the ways in which the boundaries of nation and empire have influenced the scope of British medicine in the world and as a social institution domestically. *Fit to Practice* is an institutional history of the General Council of Medical Education and Registration of the United Kingdom (GMC) and its management of the register between 1858 and 1978. As provided for in the landmark 1858 Medical Act, the register was more than a listing of doctors with approved medical qualifications; it also functioned as a common or national portal of entry into the profession for medical graduates from England, Scotland, and Ireland. The register defined the national and imperial boundaries of the jurisdiction of British medicine and membership within it, not only mediating where British medical graduates could practice medicine in the world, but also who was fit to represent British medicine domestically. As I will show, the register operated as a political instrument to preserve the privileged position of domestic medical graduates as Britain's position in the world shifted from an imperial nation-state during the course of the long nineteenth century to a member state of the European Economic Community (EEC) in the second half of the twentieth century.

This book therefore seeks to historicize British medicine within a much broader chronological and spatial framework than has customarily been the case. British medicine is a peculiar category in that it lacks a legal status—the medical degrees and diplomas awarded in the United Kingdom do not bear the phrase British medicine. Still, it occupies a distinctive political space. As early as the nineteenth century, the term *British medicine* did not refer to a specific jurisdiction per se. Rather, it referred to the multiple medical jurisdictions within the British archipelago itself—the English, Scottish, and Irish degree- and diploma-granting institutions—while superimposing an additional British identity. In practice, the centers of education and training in Edinburgh, London, and Dublin served as critical social spaces for the formation of a nascent British elite in the profession up through the midcentury.[1] At the same time, the founding of the Provincial Medical and Surgical Association in 1832 began the process of organizing nonelite practitioners outside of London. Its name change to the British Medical Association (BMA) in 1857 announced an explicit ambition to represent the interests of all medical practitioners throughout the United Kingdom.[2]

Yet the political invention of British medicine reflected the world outside of the archipelago as it did within it. In this book, I ground the making of British medicine within the historical processes of imperialism. A growing body of scholarship has demonstrated that the British "empire" not only defined the territorial boundaries of the British nation-state but also inflected the meaning of national identity and belonging domestically.[3] These effects shaped and informed the development of the medical profession throughout the twentieth century. As I have argued elsewhere, the Victorian empire provided a destination for the surplus supply of domestic medical graduates, offering preferential employment in the various state and colonial services. It also figured as a rhetorical space in the metropolitan press, which constructed British medicine as a civilizing agent in the world.[4] All of these conditions helped to define domestic graduates as "British" doctors even though they obtained their medical qualifications in England, Scotland, or Ireland.

Fit to Practice locates the place of overseas doctors of color in Britain not only within a specific set of postwar circumstances, but also in relationship to the historical invention of British medicine within the context of British imperialism. Although the medical register ostensibly masked national differences within the archipelago, the meaning of British medicine was continually contested. The contradiction yielded regular conflicts about the scope of the territorial jurisdiction of the register and the social structure of British medicine. The conflicts between the GMC and territories reflected Britain's changing political relationship to the empire. Local professions and provincial legislatures in white settler colonies or dominions pushed for greater autonomy in controlling access to their medical markets. Operating under Britain's imperial political authority, the council policed the rights of domestic medical graduates in and outside of the United Kingdom. Beginning in 1886, reciprocity, which opened the register to overseas doctors, provided a means to maintain the territorial integrity of British medicine for domestic graduates. In practice, reciprocity did not so much resolve conflict as produce another fault line of tension that revealed the politically constructed nature of British medicine. At issue was whether individual reciprocating countries and dominions were obligated to honor all of Britain's agreements and thereby open their markets to all doctors on the register. Until 1927 the GMC interpreted admission to the register broadly and enforced the right of unrestricted access for registered overseas doctors in all reciprocating countries and territories. But once Britain recognized the undivided sovereignty of dominions as independent nation-states legally in 1927 and politically in 1931, the scope of reciprocity narrowed. This shift in policy not only signaled the decline of the imperial scope of the jurisdiction of British medicine whereby any doctor on the British register could practice medicine in any reciprocating country or territory as if they were trained in the United Kingdom. Countries reciprocating with Britain were now legally entitled to limit access to their markets to British medical graduates and to deny rights of practice to doctors from other reciprocating countries or territories. It, too, established a precedent for treating overseas doctors on the register differentially.

These conflicts about where a registered doctor could practice in the world were complemented by disputes over who was fit to represent British medicine. *Fit to Practice* documents how the political process of expanding the participation of socially marginalized populations in British medicine exposed this institution's underlying inequalities, calling into question the purported meritocratic basis of membership within it. These inequalities ranged from the persistence of informal barriers to women accessing medical education and obtaining registrable qualifications, to the withdrawal of GMC recognition of Indian medical qualifications once Indians assumed greater control of medical education during the interwar period, to the imposition of quotas on the number of foreign Jewish medical refugees who were permitted to requalify in the United Kingdom on the eve of World War II.[5] It is important to note that access to the register was neither unilaterally nor indefinitely closed. Women and Jewish refugees were admitted but in limited numbers. The GMC restored recognition of Indian qualifications though on an annual or periodic basis. There is no doubt that economic concerns influenced the limited or qualified social accommodation within the profession. It is equally clear that women, colonial Indian, and Jewish refugee doctors practicing medicine under the authority of the register disrupted the identity of the profession as normatively male and white or British.[6]

At the same time, the imperative to preserve the privileged position of British doctors informed the decision to tactically open the register to overseas-trained doctors from in- and outside the Commonwealth during the exigencies of World Wars I and II. Overseas doctors provided a critical resource for medical labor. They supplemented the constrained capacity of domestic medical schools to expand and relieved some of the burden on the profession to meet the personnel needs of the military and those of the civilian population.[7] Further, the temporary nature of these wartime crises and the expectation that overseas doctors would return to their country of origin or country where they obtained their primary medical qualification moderated anxieties about opening the register to the world. But this posture toward overseas doctors would change in the postwar period.

Indeed, one of the central paradoxes of the period is Britain's continued utilization of medical labor from overseas and the growing anxiety about their presence within and without the profession. As others have noted, what changed was the fact that a significant number of these doctors were from nonwhite countries in the Commonwealth, especially India and Pakistan.[8] Even though their labor was indispensable to the delivery of health care to the nation through the network of state hospitals in the National Health Service (NHS), their presence became politically contentious. To be sure, the unprecedented size and scope of the globalization of British medicine informed the rhetoric about their medical training and professional competency. There was more to this rhetoric, though, than racism or simply defending patient safety. Britain's reliance on overseas doctors of color compelled the profession and public alike to confront the underlying contradictions of British medicine. South Asian doctors not only embodied the enmeshed boundaries of nation and empire that historically defined British medicine as a domestic profession, but these doctors also challenged whiteness as the underlying social basis of membership within it. As I will show, the GMC and the state responded to the political crisis of British medicine by redefining who was fit to practice medicine and under what conditions in the United Kingdom.

Ranging over more than a century and drawing on a variety of sources, this book charts the transformation of the world from a destination for the surplus supply of domestic medical graduates to a tactical resource for medical labor. Part 1 examines the invention of British medicine since the mid-nineteenth century. Chapter 1 covers the period between the two legislative cornerstones of British medicine: the 1858 Medical Act and its amendment in 1886. It focuses on how the social consequences and political challenges to British medicine as an exclusive imperial national profession spurred the opening of the register. In 1876, parliamentary legislation enabled women to be examined for registrable medical qualifications in Britain while provisions for reciprocity in 1886 opened the register to select territories and countries. Neither significantly affected the essential character of national medicine as white, predominately male, and overwhelmingly British. Still, the political management of the national and imperial boundaries of British medicine before and after World War I consumed more of the council's attention. As I discuss in chapter 3, a growing number of participating countries and colonies adopted local legislation to restrict access to their markets to medical graduates on the register who obtained their qualifications in the United Kingdom rather than a third country reciprocating with Britain. This narrow application of reciprocity not only challenged the council's more expansive interpretation—which presumed that all doctors on the register were entitled to the unrestricted practice of medicine—but also caused the jurisdiction of British medicine in the world to oscillate.

Chapters 2 and 4 detail the uses of reciprocity to serve the strategic interests of the imperial nation-state. Before World War I, opening the register enabled Britain to accommodate the medical preferences of nationals traveling or living abroad; forge partnerships with other imperial nation-states; and sustain the social and political connections between Britain and its far-flung territories. With the outbreak of war, Britain harnessed these political relationships to supplement its constrained capacity to produce doctors for total war. At the outbreak of war in 1914, overseas-trained doctors accounted for 10 percent; by the end of the war in 1919, they accounted for 34 percent of all admissions. Britain mobilized medical labor on an even larger scale during World War II. In addition to tapping reciprocating countries, the war cabinet promulgated a series of temporary registration orders that opened the register to doctors from allied, neutral, and belligerent countries. An underlying assumption animating the use of medical labor was the restoration of the domestic market when peacetime returned. In short, overseas-trained doctors would return home after their service. This assumption, for the most part, was borne out after World Wars I and II.

Part 2 explores the remaking of British medicine in the second half of the twentieth century. As I discuss in chapter 5, the postwar period witnessed the globalization of the domestic profession. The two routes to the register—full registration for doctors from reciprocating countries and temporary registration for doctors from nonreciprocating countries—facilitated the continuous movement of overseas doctors to Britain. This movement was unprecedented both for its size and scale and for the social characteristics of the doctors themselves. South Asian doctors were drawn to Britain for advanced hospital-based training, and their labor proved to be essential to the operation of the hospital service of the National Health Service (NHS), a major pillar of the postwar social welfare state. Even though their labor supplemented the domestic output of medical graduates, observers in- and outside of the profession increasingly viewed their presence as an existential threat to British medicine itself. Their racialized visibility revealed the breakdown of the territorial and social boundaries that had historically constructed British medicine as a domestic social institution. Growing criticism of a system of registration that privileged doctors from "new" Commonwealth countries over doctors from Europe reinforced the fictive homogeneity of British medicine while spurring increased scrutiny about the fitness of overseas doctors of color to practice medicine in the United Kingdom.

Both the GMC and the state were deeply implicated in the political problem of overseas doctors, as I show in chapters 6 and 7. The 1886 Medical Act provided for the government to extend reciprocity and the council to recognize medical qualifications in participating countries for admission to the register. Although the institutional responses of both these parties to the globalization of British medicine were different, the effect was largely the same: narrowing the terms and conditions under which overseas doctors could access the register and practice medicine. In 1974 the Conservative government led by Edward Heath retracted reciprocity from Pakistan, and a year later the council withdrew recognition from Indian medical schools. South Asian medical graduates therefore could only access the register through the highly restrictive conditions of temporary registration. These actions cast doubt on the medical training and English-language competency of South Asians and confirmed a postwar discourse that had questioned the fitness of overseas doctors of color to practice medicine. They also affirmed public anxiety about and justified increased professional surveillance of overseas doctors while reinforcing the privileged status of domestic graduates as far more accomplished. As I discuss in chapter 8, the public inquiry into the regulation of the profession, which focused among other subjects on the oversight of the register by the GMC, validated public and professional sentiment about overseas doctors of color, including those who were fully registered. Ultimately, the competency of all doctors of color remained in doubt precisely because of their discordant presence within the boundaries of a historically constructed national profession that was white, largely male, and British.

Part One

Inventing British Medicine

Chapter One

Mediating Nation and Empire in the Political Landscape of British Medicine in the World, 1858–86

Introduction

Nation and empire defined the boundaries of medicine in the United Kingdom. But these boundaries did not encompass a unified or British jurisdiction until 1858. Instead, there were informal and formal jurisdictions. University medical degrees as well as diplomas and certificates awarded by professional colleges in England, Scotland, and Ireland controlled access to medical markets in the archipelago and state-mandated medical services in the empire. The Medical Act of 1858 altered this landscape. It provided for a unified jurisdiction and a single market through the establishment of a medical register. The register, which comprised a list of practitioners who were deemed "legally qualified," operated as a common portal of entry into the medical profession for English, Irish, and Scottish medical graduates. This was only possible because university and nonuniversity licensing bodies modified their relationship with each other and the British imperial nation-state. Instead of serving their own narrow interests, they now functioned as equivalent routes to a national register. The rights enjoyed by graduates were one and the same. Their qualifications guaranteed admission to the register and, most importantly, the unrestricted right to practice medicine in the United Kingdom and the territorial empire. Of course, integration did not happen overnight. But the act created a framework for it to develop. Doctors retained their national affiliation with England, Wales, Scotland, or Ireland while adding an imperial or British identity. The combination of a common portal and a demarcated jurisdiction for the practice of medicine created the basis for a liberal imperial profession at midcentury. The scope of the authority of the British medical qualification in the world was based not necessarily on the superiority of domestic medical education per se, but rather on Britain's position as an imperial power. Any registered doctor could practice medicine wherever the Union Jack flew. The national and imperial reach of the newly formed field of British medicine therefore implicated all medical graduates and bodies in the defense and expansion of this jurisdiction.

As I will discuss in this chapter, admission to the register reinforced the social character of the profession as a space for white men. Women faced formal barriers to medical education and licensing examinations in the United Kingdom. These barriers, which were actively policed, had the effect of naturalizing the social identity of the profession as male. This was similarly the case for the racialization of British medicine as white. The legal relationship between domestic medical qualifications and eligibility for positions in the imperial services virtually ensured that representatives of the empire were white and male. Even in territories in the nonwhite dependent empire where instruction in western medicine was available, this instruction reinforced British rule. Such training produced a subordinate medical labor force that supplemented British doctors while buttressing the racial hierarchy of the empire.

The Invention of British Medicine: The General Council of Medical Education and Registration, 1858–70

Before the passage of the 1858 Medical Act, there were multiple portals of entry into the medical markets of the United Kingdom of Great Britain and Ireland. Some twenty-one self-governing bodies—that is, universities, corporate professional colleges, and the Archbishop of Canterbury—offered individual degrees, diplomas and licenses, and certificates on their own terms in the three divisions of the archipelago: England and Wales, Ireland, and Scotland. These qualifications aligned with the traditional legal orders of medicine. These included apothecaries, who compounded drugs; surgeons, who excised disease; and physicians, who treated illness. These qualifications not only subjected recipients to the control of the granting medical authority, but they also entitled members to legal rights and institutional privileges such as the right to practice throughout the empire or obtain employment in the army, navy, and East Indian Company or on slave ships.[1]

The institutionally decentralized nature of medicine yielded a variety of standards of medical training and practice, which reflected a much broader landscape of medical pluralism. Conflict and competition animated this market as corporate bodies defended or sought to open up monopolistic privileges. The seemingly neat traditional legal orders of medicine did not remain unaffected. Designated roles began to blur into a new hybrid—the general medical practitioner. Neither a physician nor a surgeon, the practitioner treated patients and dispensed medicine with a primary qualification from the College of Surgeons. The Apothecaries Act of 1815 provided a de facto credential for the general practitioner. The act mandated that surgeons hold a license from the Apothecaries' Society of England as a condition to engage in general practice. This act is noteworthy for another reason: it represented the only major piece of legislation affecting entry into the profession until the passage of the Medical Act in 1858.[2]

As scholars have demonstrated, the 1858 Medical Act was an imperfect milestone in the process of creating a national medical profession.[3] The act was permissive and did not explicitly define or privilege any particular theoretical basis of medicine. Still, it enabled practitioners to designate themselves as "legally qualified" in the eyes of the state and thereby publicly distinguish themselves from nonqualified practitioners. This designation depended on the possession of at least one qualification—a diploma, degree, or license in medicine, surgery, or apothecary from a schedule of nineteen university and nonuniversity licensing bodies. The medical register complemented this "common" or national portal. The register furnished the public with a list of "legally qualified" doctors who voluntarily added their names. Regardless of where a practitioner obtained his qualification, all registered doctors were now entitled by law to practice medicine, surgery, or both medicine and surgery in the United Kingdom, including Britain's territorial empire. As a group, they were permitted to sue and collect fees in a court of law; sign death certificates; and enjoyed exemption from jury service, inquests, and county militias. Only registered doctors were eligible for posts that either were funded publicly or were associated with chartered organizations. These entities ranged from army and naval services or passenger service to friendly or mutual aid societies, asylums, and poor law workhouses, among others.[4]

Regulating participation in the profession was the charge of the GMC. Administratively, the GMC consisted of three branch councils: one each for England, Ireland, and Scotland. While each council was empowered to appoint its own registrar to maintain its list of qualified doctors, treasurer, and clerks, the English branch functioned as the administrative center for the management of the consolidated medical register. The governing body of the GMC consisted of twenty-five members: nineteen represented university and nonuniversity licensing bodies and six were crown appointees (see table 1.1). Led by an elected president, the council was the policymaking body and delegated its activities to an executive committee, standing committees, and ad hoc committees as needed. The principle of majority rule on all matters before the council grounded collective responsibility on consensus. No

Table 1.1. Institutional representatives on the General Medical Council of Medical Education and Registration, 1858

Country	Institution
England	Royal College of Physicians
	Royal College of Surgeons of England
	Apothecaries' Society of London
	University of Oxford
	University of Cambridge
	University of Durham
	University of London
Scotland	College of Physicians of Edinburgh
	University of Edinburgh
	The College of Surgeons of Edinburgh
	The Faculty of Physicians and Surgeons of Glasgow
	University of Aberdeen
	University of Glasgow
	University of Saint Andrews
Ireland	King's and Queen's College of Ireland
	Royal College of Surgeons of Ireland
	Apothecaries' Hall of Ireland
	University of Ireland, Dublin
	Queen's University in Ireland

Source: Section 4; 46 & 47 Medical Act c. 90.

one particular group—whether university or nonuniversity licensing bodies or crown appointees—could unilaterally dictate the conditions of entry into a national profession or participation in a national market.[5]

Even as this structure created a space for British medicine within local institutions, it simultaneously embedded the GMC in a set of political relationships that circumscribed its power to regulate the profession. The licensing bodies, whose representatives formed a majority of the council membership, retained their corporate autonomy, including control over their individual curricula and examinations. Collectively, they conferred twenty medical, surgical, and midwifery licenses for a grand total of fifty-one possible qualifications (see tables 1.2 and 1.3). These independent points of entry translated into differing standards. Since each qualification entitled the bearer to admission to the register, practitioners were not required to complement their single competency with a second. At most,

Table 1.2. Qualifications conferred by the medical authorities in the United Kingdom

Medical authorities that granted qualifications in both medicine and surgery
Royal College of Physicians of London
University of Cambridge
University of Durham
University of London
University of Edinburgh
University of Aberdeen
University of Glasgow
University of St. Andrews
University of Dublin
Queen's University in Ireland
Medical authorities that granted qualifications in surgery only
Royal College of Surgeons of England
Royal College of Surgeons of Edinburgh
Faculty of Physicians and Surgeons of Glasgow
Royal College of Surgeons in Ireland
Medical authorities that granted qualifications in medicine only
Royal College of Physicians of Edinburgh
King's and Queen's College of Physicians in Ireland
University of Oxford
Apothecaries' Hall of Ireland
Medical authorities that granted qualifications in midwifery only
King's and Queen's College of Physicians in Ireland
Royal College of Surgeons of England
Royal College of Surgeons of Ireland

Source: Return on Qualifications Conferred Several Medical Authorities, appendix no. 4 in *Select Committee on the Medical Amendment Act* (1878–79), 343.

Table 1.3. Qualifications conferred by university and nonuniversity licensing bodies before 1886

Country	Institution	Qualifications conferred
England	Royal College of Physicians	Fellow, Licentiate, extra Licentiate
	Royal College of Surgeons of England	Fellow, Member, Licentiate
	Apothecaries' Society of London	Licentiate
	University of Oxford	Doctor, Bachelor, Licentiate, Master in Medicine or Surgery
	University of Cambridge	Doctor, Bachelor, Licentiate, Master in Medicine or Surgery
	University of Durham	Doctor, Bachelor, Licentiate, Master in Medicine or Surgery
	University of London	Doctor, Bachelor, Licentiate, Master in Medicine or Surgery
Ireland	King's and Queen's College of Ireland	Doctor, Bachelor, Licentiate, Master
	Royal College of Surgeons of Ireland	Fellow or Licentiate
	Apothecaries' Hall of Ireland	Licentiate
	University of Ireland, Dublin	Doctor, Bachelor, Licentiate, Master in Medicine or Surgery
	Queen's University in Ireland	Doctor, Bachelor, Licentiate, Master in Medicine or Surgery
Scotland	Royal College of Physicians of Edinburgh	Fellow, Licentiate
	Royal College of Surgeons of Edinburgh	Fellow, Licentiate
	Faculty of Physicians and Surgeons of Glasgow	Fellow, Licentiate
	University of Edinburgh	Doctor, Bachelor, Licentiate, Master in Medicine or Surgery
	University of Aberdeen	Doctor, Bachelor, Licentiate, Master in Medicine or Surgery
	University of Glasgow	Doctor, Bachelor, Licentiate, Master in Medicine or Surgery
	University of Saint Andrews	Doctor, Bachelor, Licentiate, Master in Medicine or Surgery

Source: List of Qualifications Registerable in the "Medical Register," appendix 11, paper 10 in *Select Committee on the Medical Amendment Act* (1878–79), 414.

provision in the legislation only encouraged two nonuniversity licensing colleges or bodies to conjoin or "unite or cooperate in conducting the examinations required for examinations required for qualifications to be registered under this Act." Although conjoint examinations did form, the single qualified practitioners on the register remained a concern that would spur efforts to amend legislation throughout the century.[6]

The duties reserved to the GMC for oversight in education underscored the supremacy of the licensing bodies. The GMC was authorized to request information regarding the courses of study as well as to assign visitors to observe and report on examinations. It was not empowered to refuse to register or suspend a scheduled qualification. At most, it could recommend changes to the curriculum or examinations, which were left to the individual licensing bodies to adopt. Further, the capacity of the GMC to take the initiative was constrained by the limited nature of its funding. The act empowered the council to impose a one-time registration fee at admission. These fees were collected at the branch councils in England, Scotland, and Ireland and used to defray the expenses of the GMC associated with the "keeping, printing, and publishing of the register for the United Kingdom." The government provided no subventions.[7]

Moreover, the medical council was constitutionally subordinate to the Privy Council, an intergovernmental body that oversaw all regulatory bodies that were incorporated by Royal Charter. The Privy Council's oversight ranged from approval of bylaw revisions, to new regulations and their implementation, to disciplinary decisions affecting corporate members or membership. With reference to discipline, the medical council could only recommend the revocation of a scheduled qualification, but it was up to the Privy Council to give the recommendation effect in an Order in Council.[8] While the Medical Act outlined the place of the GMC within the larger state apparatus, its independence placed it in a politically tenuous position. Mandated to protect the public, the GMC was a nonpartisan body and therefore lacked a base of political support like the BMA or the nineteen licensing bodies.[9] The council could only look to the government to advance any amending legislation to the Medical Act, or conversely react to its initiatives, which was typically the case. The support of the government was rarely guaranteed and was subject to multiple imperatives, including (among others) party interests, the state's role in society, and external relations. For this reason, the posture of the GMC tended to be reactive and contingent on the receptivity of power centers both within and outside of the government and the state.

The Register as a Gateway to the Empire

British medicine developed hand in hand with British imperialism. In practice, the GMC facilitated this relationship. Its largely passive role reflected its subordinate position to the executive committee and the institutional autonomy of the licensing bodies that comprised the majority of the council. The 1858 Medical Act neither required medical graduates to add their names to the medical register nor granted registrants a monopoly on the practice of medicine. Instead, the state linked the possession of a medical qualification and employment to its personnel needs as its role in society and the world expanded. This connection increasingly yoked the fortunes of British medicine to the growth of the bureaucratic and territorial state. Indeed, the passage of the act took place against the backdrop of legislative initiatives that sought to mitigate the health effects of industrialization and urbanization. Factory, poor law, prison, and passenger vessel reform generated a growing number of public medical appointments charged with addressing the needs of those who were deemed vulnerable to accidents and illness or bearers of disease and threats to public health.[10] Furthermore, the expansion of the Victorian empire increased the demand for qualified practitioners to deliver medical care to the charges of the imperial state or other consumers of medicine. These charges ranged from imperial servants who served in the army and navy, government personnel, and subjects of the colonial state to laborers, migrants, and sailors who circulated through the empire and between the metropole and the periphery. By the end of the century, the total number of positions in the principal state services (army, India, and navy) and in the colonial services in territories ruled by Britain employed an estimated 2,500 practitioners or 10 percent of the domestic profession.[11]

Imperial Service and the Making of the Racial Boundaries of British Medicine

The prescribed university and nonuniversity licensing medical qualifications awarded by domestic institutions and state service helped cement an imperial profession that was effectively, if not exclusively, white and male.[12] No formal rules barred nonwhite colonial subjects from medical training in the United Kingdom or appointments in the state services, but the educational requirements of admission to a university or nonuniversity licensing body in the metropole for all practical purposes limited the number of colonial subjects to a relatively privileged minority that could afford it or were sponsored by the imperial state, a colonial government, or missionaries.[13] Even for western-educated Indians, the opportunity costs—such as passage fees and living expenses—were significant obstacles. The earliest Indians to qualify in Britain were subsidized by the East India Company. In 1842 Soorjo Coomar Goodeve Chuckerbutty, B. N. Bose, D. N. Bose, and G. C. Seal were admitted to University College and became members of the Royal College of Surgeons in 1848.[14] But these were the exceptions. The vast majority of

Indians who sought and secured western training in India comprised both a captive market for the medical colleges and a pool of labor for the colonial state. During the era of East India Company rule, training institutions were established in Bombay and Calcutta to provide the Indian army with supplemental medical labor such as native subassistant surgeons, dressers, and apothecaries. Although these institutions were later taken over or supplanted by Grant Medical College and the Medical School, their purpose remained largely unchanged.[15]

Also unchanged was the subordinate status of medical graduates of these and other colleges. They were ineligible to enter the Indian Medical Service (IMS), the principal medical service of the government of India. Beginning in 1855, the India Office adopted an entry examination that was public and competitive. These attributes reflected a Victorian focus on testing as a far more equitable basis for awarding government posts than the exercise of patronage. But this condition substituted a new type of privilege even as it sought to replace an older one. After the 1858 Act only candidates who held registerable qualifications from a domestic university or professional college were eligible to sit for the examination, which was held exclusively in London. This condition closed off the IMS to Indian medical graduates since the GMC did not begin to recognize Indian qualifications until 1896.[16] Before then, the career horizon of these graduates was limited to service in the provincial medical department or private practice. This tiered career track for British and Indian graduates reproduced the racial hierarchy of colonial rule: Indian subordination to a white British male representative of the colonial state. Between 1855 and 1914, only fifty-five Indian doctors joined the IMS. By 1920 nearly one thousand Indian graduates served in the provincial services as assistant surgeons and four times that number as subassistant surgeons.[17]

Until the 1860s, medical training in Britain was relatively inaccessible for nonwhite colonial subjects in West Africa. One of the earliest was William Fergusson, a mulatto born into a merchant family in the West Indies. Following a common practice among privileged white West Indians, Fergusson traveled to Scotland where he received his diploma from the Royal College of Surgeons in 1813 and was commissioned as an officer of the Royal African Corps of the British Army in 1813.[18] In the absence of a pool of trained medical labor to supplement British military personnel, the War Department in 1854 launched an experimental initiative. It agreed to subsidize the medical education of mission-educated West Africans in exchange for military service. Underlying this initiative was the assumption that African bodies could better tolerate the tropical environment that was known as the "white man's grave." Of the four who were ultimately selected, Samuel Campbell, William Davis, and James Beale Horton qualified in 1858 and were commissioned in 1859. Upon their return to Africa, they were posted to the Gold Coast, which was notorious for high troop mortality and morbidity and meager opportunities for private practice. Their leave privileges were far less generous than those granted to their white counterparts. It was the exception rather than the rule when they were promoted to responsible positions over whites.[19] For some medical officers, even these informal markers of racial bias were insufficient. "One medical officer is said to have had it in contemplation," reported an article in *The Lancet*, "even to resign his commission rather than subject himself to the passive but not less harassing annoyances to which he felt exposed through the appointment of a native surgeon."[20] This departmental initiative was not extended beyond the initial cohort.

In the meantime, a dozen or more West Africans began self-funding their medical education in the United Kingdom. They returned to build their careers by holding positions in the colonial medical services in the Gambia, Gold Coast, Lagos, and Sierra Leone.[21] These positions afforded a measure of status within colonial society as well as opportunities for building a private practice among European fee-paying patients and contracting services with trading companies. Their medical qualifications, however, were no protection against the vagaries of bias. Using their discretionary authority in the appointment process, British officials in the Colonial Office in London and colonial governments engaged in a de facto "white only" policy. This policy was not inflexible however. When no white male doctor could be recruited or retained, a nonwhite was generally found serviceable.[22] In spite of this policy, the effectiveness of West African doctors in the service was recognized by colonial officers and patients alike. But the promotion of Sierra Leonean John Farrell Easmon as chief medical officer of the Gold Coast was, again, the exception rather than the rule. By 1902 the "white only" de facto policy was formalized with the regional consolidation of the colonial medical services into the West African Medical Service. Africans as well as Indians with registerable degrees were prohibited from employment in the service.[23]

The relationship between imperial service and the possession of a registerable degree created an explicit link between British medicine and the empire. This link was hardly exceptional given the historical nexus between licensing bodies and the empire, but it additionally reflected the active participation of the profession in the expansion of the authority of the bureaucratic and imperial state. What was distinctive about the register as a gateway to imperial service was the way in which it defined the social boundaries of membership in British medicine. The requirement to qualify in the United Kingdom established a steep hurdle for most colonial subjects in India and West Africa. Success did not fundamentally alter the racial hierarchy of British medicine in the periphery. In India the existence of a growing number of graduates from provincial medical colleges created an underclass of medical labor that supplemented the British-dominated IMS. Similarly,

West Africans who qualified and entered the colonial services of the region encountered de facto and formal policies that either marginalized them or ensured their subordinate status in relation to white British doctors.

Negotiating the Tensions of Nation and Empire within the Territorial Boundaries of British Medicine

The empire served not only as an extension of the authority of the Victorian state, but also as a vast new market for British medicine. Several scholars have documented the movement of medical graduates after the Medical Act to British territories, particularly those dominated by white settlers.[24] These doctors, like others who obtained appointments in the imperial or colonial medical services, responded to a number of factors. In constrained markets like Scotland and Ireland, medical graduates were drawn to opportunities in growing colonial societies such as Canada, Cape Colony, and Victoria among others as the century unfolded. Neither were English medical graduates immune to the push of underemployment and the pull of opportunity. Given the role of the empire as a destination for the surplus population of British doctors, any change that circumscribed the unrestricted rights of domestic graduates to practice in the empire or opened the domestic market to colonial or foreign-trained doctors was greeted with skepticism, if not outright opposition.

Almost from its inception, the council confronted challenges to the authority of British medicine. This was not a surprise. Even though the Medical Act charged the GMC to regulate the profession, this did not mean that its authority was unquestioned or that a consensus existed about who could practice medicine and where within its jurisdiction.[25] Opening the register to overseas doctors was a recurrent subject that the council weighed in on, but only at the request of the president of the Privy Council or a cabinet member. Shortly before the fall of the liberal government in 1866, Home Secretary Sir George Grey announced his intention to introduce legislation to address defects in the existing act. The council welcomed provisions put forward in this proposed legislation that would mandate two qualifications or the passing of a conjoint examination as a condition of registration. They hoped that this change would promote consistency in the content of medical education while reducing the number of qualifications that were registrable.

However the council also raised concerns about a proposed clause regarding the automatic admission of foreign and colonial medical graduates to the register. Grey's bill authorized any principal secretary of state to recognize the qualifications of foreign and colonial institutions for purposes of registration. This provision placed foreign and colonial university and nonuniversity licensing bodies on the same footing as those in the United

Kingdom while at the same time expanding the territorial portals of entry into the profession to include Europe and the empire. While the proposed clause empowered the council to exempt individuals from the provisions of the act on a case-by-case basis, it also significantly diluted the power of the council in managing the jurisdiction of British medicine.

On behalf of the GMC executive committee, the council president sought a meeting with Grey to discuss their concerns about the act. But the meeting would be overtaken by wider currents in national politics. The liberal government fell and Grey was replaced by Sir Spencer Walpole of the new Conservative government. Walpole was soon succeeded by Gathorne Hardy in May 1867. Regardless of the political orientation of the government, deputations from the council received noncommittal responses or, at best, conditional support. "Courteous reception, an attentive, and apparently a willing audience, listening to a rather long statement and to many arguments, ending with an expression of profound regret that the pressure of business would not allow of medical legislation in the present session," was how council president George Burrows summarized the meetings.[26] Walpole refused to modify Grey's proposed bill because it was the work of the previous liberal government and only pledged not to oppose the unchanged bill if introduced as a private members bill.[27]

These conditions were not well received by members of the council. For Andrew Wood of Edinburgh University, the council was being "asked to consent to a measure which would virtually subvert the power of the Council." The danger of extending reciprocal privileges without sufficient information was highlighted by the example of the United States, where medical degrees were very loosely regulated. "The regulations were so different, that the term university in many cases did not mean the same as in England. In America . . . any two or three persons might combine, and, having obtained recognition by the state, might call themselves a university; and, if laboring under that very common disease of impecuniosity, might seek a remedy in the granting of degrees on conditions would not be recognized here. The Council would be exposing themselves to great danger if they accepted Mr. Walpole's proposal."[28] The council pressed its case with the new home secretary Gathorne Hardy.[29]

The government's position was unyielding. Recognizing this political reality, Sir George Paget, chair of the committee on the amendment of the Medical Act and representative of the Royal College of Surgeons, put forward a compromise proposal. His proposal sought to preserve the authority of the council to regulate admission to the register without either sharing this responsibility with the government or extending reciprocal privileges to specific institutions outside of the United Kingdom. To this end, Paget tied council recognition of the equivalence of overseas qualifications to those conferred in the United Kingdom. First, such diplomas and degrees had to legally entitle the holder "to practice medicine and surgery in the countries where they have been granted." Second, the council had to "receive satisfactory evidence that those degrees or diplomas, or licenses to practice, have been granted after a course of study and examinations such as to secure the possession by persons obtaining them of the requisite knowledge and skill for the practice of their profession."[30]

James Syme, professor of clinical surgery at Edinburgh University, captured the mood of resignation. "It was evidently the desire of the Government to admit foreign graduates to the Register. Should then, the Council remain inactive, or do something in the matter?" Syme added that the "latter course was the proper one; and that Dr. Paget's proposal was the best that could be adopted." Even though the proposal stopped far short of granting reciprocal privileges to foreign institutions, broadening access to the register undermined the council's aspiration for a unitary national portal based on consistent standards of education and training that were subject to review and inspection. In seconding Paget's proposal, Caesar Hawkins, the representative for the Royal College of Surgeons of England, insisted that all foreign graduates be examined in the United Kingdom. Dominic Corrigan (Queen's University Ireland) went even further. He objected to "dealing with the colonial universities in the same clause as foreign universities, of which the council could know little or nothing, while they could have no difficulty in gaining correct information regarding colonies bodies." Corrigan feared that the council would be compelled to register any licensed qualification. He therefore moved an amendment that established an even higher threshold for foreign graduates to surmount before being admitted to the register. Under his amendment, all holders of foreign degrees were required to sit and pass an examination by one of the scheduled licensing bodies. In the event that they refused to accommodate a foreign graduate to sit for an examination, the council would be empowered "to register the holders of such foreign diplomas without such examination."[31]

Risdon Bennett, who represented the Royal College of Physicians of London, sympathized with Corrigan's concerns, although he opposed Corrigan's amendment out of expediency. "The question was not what was best to be done, but what must be done." If anything, the proposed differential treatment would exacerbate the insecurity faced by British medical graduates on the continent. In support of Paget's proposal, Bennett added the potential for improvements in the relation between registered doctors and host countries. He volunteered that "many English practitioners residing abroad had to submit to hardships, unless they could obtain a license of the country in which they were residing. He had in his hand a letter from a medical gentleman on the continent, who complained that nothing had been done here to ensure to persons in his condition the same privileges as were enjoyed in England by the holders of foreign diplomas." In the end,

Corrigan's amendment failed. Paget's proposal passed. This outcome certainly reflected the changing posture of the council toward doctors trained outside of the United Kingdom, but it still lacked the legal authority to recognize doctors with foreign medical qualifications for purpose of admission to the register. In the meantime, doctors trained in foreign countries or the colonies could practice medicine in the United Kingdom or the empire, but they lacked the protections and rights of a registered doctor. Enabling legislation would have to wait nearly two decades, when political circumstances mobilized Parliament to act.[32]

In the meantime, the council resisted any real or perceived infringement on the right of British-registered doctors to practice medicine in colonial markets. In the spring of 1868, the Colonial Secretary the Duke of Buckingham introduced legislation in the House of Lords to amend the Medical Act.[33] The purpose of the Medical Practitioners (Colonial) Bill was to recognize the authority of colonial legislatures and designated medical bodies to regulate access to the local medical market in the empire. Buckingham's bill was in response to a request from representatives of Ontario and British Columbia who sought to check the growing presence of unlicensed or irregular practitioners from other provinces in their medical markets. In seeking to strengthen local control, the bill reflected recent imperial legislation that sought to reconcile responsible government with imperial control. The 1867 British North America Act, which created the federated dominion of Canada, acknowledged the authority of provinces over their internal affairs. But there were limits to this authority. The Colonial Validity Act provided that the imperial Parliament could review colonial legislation that might be in conflict with metropolitan interests. In such cases, Britain retained the power to hold inoperative any law that was deemed to be "repugnant," discriminatory, or otherwise superseded imperial statutes.[34]

The "Bill to Amend the Law relating to Medical Practitioners in the Colonies" sparked a heated struggle for control of the practice of medicine in the empire. As the Bill passed its second reading, Buckingham was subject to public and private appeals to withdraw or revise it. An editorial in the *Medical Times and Gazette* objected that "medical Practitioners who have placed their names on the Imperial Register with the intention of practicing in the colonies may reasonably complain that they have been deprived of the privileges which they bought when they paid their money in Soho-square." While acknowledging "the natural tendency of colonial institutions to become in time independent of those of the mother county," the editorial warned of the consequences to British medicine should the Bill become law. "If the British registered Practitioner is not permitted to exercise his Profession in the colonies without examination by or payment to the local boards, there can be no pretext for admitting the possessors of colonial degrees to the Imperial Register without subjecting them to some further proof of their fitness." The bias in favor of colonial degrees over foreign ones seemed poised to end as well. "Should this Act pass, the relations of the Medical Council to the colonial Universities and examining boards will be greatly simplified. There will, in fact, be no reason for placing these bodies in a different category from that of the American and European Universities and Colleges," said the *Medical Times and Gazette.*[35]

Deputations from the GMC and the BMA met with the colonial secretary in April. Alluding to the exchange between the Home Office and the council regarding the admission of colonial and foreign medical graduates to the register, Burrow reminded Buckingham of the role of the council in regulating admission to the register as well as previously stalled legislative efforts to relax admission for colonial and foreign graduates. Citing ignorance of the Home Office correspondence, Buckingham conceded the potential for "hardship" and agreed to revise the Bill. The revised language in the subsequent legislation accommodated British graduates as an editorial in the *British Medical Journal* declared[36]: "This shall retain the privileges of the British graduates, and gives to the colonies the right of making a colonial register (which is very necessary), but binds them to accept the certificate of British registration as a title of colonial registration. The objects of the Council, the Association, and the profession have thus been fully accomplished by the intervention of the deputations, and the high and intelligent sense of justice which the Colonial Secretary manifested on the occasion."[37]

Even though the Medical Act created a single jurisdiction and medical market for registered doctors, the GMC struggled to defend them. Both cabinet secretaries and the government pushed for legislation to open the register to foreign graduates or circumscribe the rights of registered doctors to practice medicine in colonial markets. These bills did not become law. The preservation of the preferential rights of registered doctors in the 1868 Medical Amendment Act following a campaign led by the BMA and the GMC underscored the emergence of British medicine as a political interest domestically and in the empire.

Gendering the Boundaries of British Medicine: Woman Doctors and Foreign Medical Degrees

While the 1868 Medical Amendment Act preserved the advantage of registered doctors in the empire, the admission of doctors with foreign qualifications to the register remained a contentious issue. This was particularly the case in reference to women who earned foreign medical degrees. Their demand to be admitted to the register challenged both the gendered and territorial boundaries of British medicine. The very legislation that invented British medicine codified male privilege in medicine. All nineteen university and nonuniversity bodies that awarded registrable qualifications were closed to women. In practice, they neither were permitted to attend medical schools or sit for professional or licensing examinations. In 1870 only two women had in fact been admitted to the register—Elizabeth Blackwell and Elizabeth Garrett Anderson. These exceptional cases underscored the exclusionary nature of British medicine. Elizabeth Blackwell received her medical education at the Geneva Medical School in New York, which promptly denied admission to women after she graduated in 1849. Under the liberal grandfather clause of the 1858 Medical Act, she was admitted to the register in 1859. By contrast, Elizabeth Garrett Anderson was admitted to the register in 1865 after qualifying in the United Kingdom. She circumvented barriers by taking advantage of the multiple portals of entry to the register. In 1860 Middlesex Hospital denied her admission to medical school. Rather than seeking education abroad, she studied privately in preparation for licensure. London University and the Royal College of Physician and Surgeons refused to permit her to sit for their examinations. The Society of Apothecaries—one of the least prestigious nonuniversity licensing bodies—agreed. She passed and was admitted to the register.[38]

Edinburgh University was the exception among universities in 1869 in allowing women to matriculate. But this was by no means a certain route to the register. The university agreed to permit Sophia Jex-Blake and three other women to study medicine, yet they faced obstacles in virtually every aspect of their education. They were segregated from male students in class and faced hazing by them outside of class. It took three years of political mobilizing and legal action to secure access to the Royal Infirmary for mandatory clinical instruction. While Jex-Blake and the other women medical students enjoyed some support from male members of the medical faculty, opponents used their influence on the faculty and in the university senate to disqualify them from sitting for the preliminary and first professional examinations. Even though the university admitted women students, the University Council proved to be unwilling to assure them a degree, preferring instead to provide women graduates "certificates of proficiency." It was only after Jex-Blake prevailed in a July 1872 suit—later upheld on appeal—that the university agreed to award degrees to women graduates in medicine. In hopes of ensuring consistency among universities, liberal members of Parliament, William Cowper-Temple and Russell Gurney, proposed legislation in January 1874 to enable Scottish universities to admit and grant degrees to women. The bill was defeated.[39]

Cowper-Temple subsequently introduced the Foreign Degrees Bill in February in 1875. His bill mandated that the council recognize for full registration foreign degrees from specific universities in Leipzig, Berne, Zurich, and the École de Medicine in Paris.[40] The bill was clearly designed to open up the register to women graduates. As the Edinburgh experience made clear, the admission of women to the register was subject to discretion. Requalification through a nonuniversity licensing body was another option for women, though this route had not been tested since Elizabeth Anderson. This was, in fact, the only means for foreign medical graduates to obtain some credit for their medical education abroad while completing mandated training in the United Kingdom. Since continental schools were relatively more open, a growing number of women sought out training on the Continent. However, unlike men who had been qualified abroad, none of the women who received medical training on the Continent during this period sought requalification in the United Kingdom. This was most likely because access to crucial anatomical courses and clinical instruction in a hospital setting was closed off to them in Britain.

For its part, the council tacitly considered foreign degrees and the admission of women in medicine as separate issues. Reflecting support within and outside of Parliament for opening up the medical profession to women, the lord president of the Privy Council solicited the views of the GMC.[41] Edinburgh professor William Turner, who ultimately refused Jex-Blake's request to be admitted to his anatomy class, chaired an ad hoc committee that produced a compromise report. It raised reservations about accommodating women within medical schools but stopped short of endorsing the legal exclusion of women. "Instead of medicine offering more facilities and less difficulties for women than other professions, the Medical Council believe, that as the whole question is looked into, there will be found peculiar hindrances, moral and physical, to the successful pursuit of medicine by women." Because the bill carried with it the assumption that women could practice medicine, Turner's ad hoc committee regarded the Cowper Temple Bill as flawed. The chief reason given by the committee was their concern about the differential treatment of men and women. "The Council cannot approve of a measure intended to confer on women the privilege of registering certain foreign degrees, from which, under Clause XLVI of the Medical Act, men are debarred, and over the education and examination for which the Medical Council have no means of exercising that supervisions and control to which all licensing bodies of this country, whether universities or medical corporations, are subjected."[42] This rationale captured the social contradictions contained within British medicine. By 1868 the council had embraced opening the register to foreign medical graduates. But in rejecting the Cowper-Temple Bill, it defended the continuation of male privilege in the name of defending the territorial boundaries of national medicine.

Cowper-Temple's bill went down in defeat. While protecting male privilege was part of the reason, the matter of admitting foreign medical graduates was undoubtedly another. It is likely for this reason that the GMC was far more accommodating to a bill proposed by Russell Gurney. Gurney's bill proposed to extend to all licensing bodies the power to admit women candidates to their examinations. But the council agreed not to oppose the bill subject to two conditions. First, the bill could not mandate but only enable the admission of women to professional examinations. The second condition was that women could not participate in the actual administration of examinations, thereby reinforcing the hierarchy of male power and female subordination in medicine.[43] Although Gurney's bill passed in 1876, British medicine remained largely unchanged. To be sure, the 1874 establishment of the London School of Medicine for Women (LSMW) opened up opportunities for medical education in part to provide medical missionaries for India.[44] The combination of access to the wards of the Royal Free Hospital and the opening of University of London degrees to students regardless of sex in 1877 increased the number of women on the register. Still, students who passed through LSMW accounted for 90 percent of women doctors on the register by 1890. This distinction underscores the narrow portal of entry to the profession for women (see table 1.4).[45]

Defending British Medicine by Expanding its Boundaries: The Making of the Medical Amendment Act, 1886

The increasing vulnerability of registered British doctors to differential treatment in jurisdictions outside of the United Kingdom spurred the council and Parliament to adopt a mechanism that provided overseas-trained doctors regulated access to the medical market of imperial Britain while affording British doctors the legal right to practice medicine abroad. Building on the eighteenth-century tradition of the grand tour, British nationals in growing numbers in the nineteenth century visited the continent for study, travel, and health restoration. British doctors were no different. A steady stream of doctors visited Paris and other urban centers of medicine to learn from eminent clinicians, who pioneered the linking of visible symptoms of disease to underlying pathological disorders and later became therapeutic innovators.[46] Women formed part of this movement to France. Still other doctors regarded the growth in travel for health restoration on the continent as an economic opportunity. Reflecting these trends, France and Italy granted conditional rights to foreign doctors to practice medicine in order to engage in study or treat nationals.

Yet, the place of British doctors in host countries became more contingent as local national professions sought to impose stricter conditions on access to the medical market. As Julie Fette has shown, the profession in France increasingly pushed for restrictive conditions on all foreign doctors as an effort to consolidate the social status and economic rewards of French medicine.[47] In May 1876, Roger Marvaise introduced a bill in the French Chamber of Deputies that proposed raising the credentialing threshold for

Table 1.4. Women on the Medical Register, 1871–1921

Year	Number on register
1871	2
1881	25
1891	100
1901	200
1911	600
1912	1,500
1913	3,300
1915	7,520
1917	12,596

Source: Stacey, *Regulating British Medicine*, 22, table 3.1.

foreign practitioners to practice medicine.[48] Under existing law, foreign nationals were allowed to practice medicine subject only to the permission of the minister of public instruction and without additional study and examination. Citing abuses such as unqualified doctors practicing medicine or cultivating practice under the pretense of study and research, Marvaise's bill mandated that all such practitioners in the future would have to complete their medical education and pass a professional examination in France as a condition to practicing medicine legally. In truth, the mandates of the bill strongly resembled the custom and practice in Britain, where foreign graduates could only be admitted to the register if they requalified, and those who were unqualified could practice as unregistered practitioners, but without legal protections. Unlike the British situation, if Marvaise's bill became law, all foreign doctors who failed to comply would be subject to a fine up to 1,000 francs and six months imprisonment.[49]

Requesting an official British protest to the French government, Wilson Fox, a fellow of the Royal College of Physicians and the Royal Society, alerted the Earl of Derby to the implications of the bill for nationals who sought treatment at health resorts in France and its territories that were run by British doctors. These residents or visitors to the Francophone world were among the more affluent members of British society. He warned that "invalids who resort to various places in France, and have hitherto counted upon the assistance of English medical men resident there" would be affected, and he noted the likely adverse economic consequence to "winter resorts as

Pau, Nice, Cannes, Mentone, Hyeres, and Algiers" in the event that British doctors were discouraged or prohibited from practicing on British nationals. While the French minister was prepared to consider the official concerns raised by the bill, he also requested a statement of the law and customs that related to foreign doctors in the United Kingdom. The Foreign Office requested the views of the GMC on the place of English and other foreign practitioners in France and the position of foreign practitioners practicing in England.[50]

In the meantime, the French dispute amplified concerns about the status of degrees or diplomas awarded in the empire. Writing on behalf of licentiates and graduates of the Universities of Calcutta, Madras, and Bombay in 1877, Joseph Fayrer, president of the London-based India Office Medical Board, requested that their qualifications entitle graduates to automatic admission to the British medical register. As the controversy over Canadian qualifications in the late 1860s revealed, colonial graduates did not have standing in the United Kingdom as registered doctors. In response to Fayrer's request and to Marvais's proposed bill, the committee on medical acts implicitly acknowledged as much. To resolve these anomalies, the committee proposed three recommendations. The first would entitle qualifications granted in the empire legal recognition in the United Kingdom. The second proposed the creation of a designated section within the register for "foreigners practicing in the United Kingdom with qualifications granted in foreign countries entitling them to practice in those countries." Another provision provided the council with the discretionary power to "cause to be registered in the section of the Register such qualifications as it may in its discretion judge to be reasonable guarantees of professional skill."[51]

The council's discussion of the report highlighted continuing tensions in reconciling the boundaries of nation and empire. Alluding to reports that local laws required foreign practitioners to pass an examination, Wood hoped that opening the register would promote better relations within the empire. He noted "an act of justice towards the colonies would lead them to do justice to British practitioners."[52] Corrigan demurred, motioning to remove the provision for a separate list for colonial practitioners, which he described as creating a distinction of an "invidious character." "When colonial practitioners were put on the Register, they would be entitled to all the privileges and immunities of ordinary registered practitioners. To place them in a separate section would indicate that they were inferior. If they were received at all, they should be received into the enjoyment of full rights, as in every respect qualified." Others defended the list as a compromise between opening the register to practitioners and the practical limits of the council's oversight over medical education outside of the United Kingdom. Simon, chair of the committee, spoke against Corrigan's motion. "The reason for proposing a separate Register was that colonial degrees were in a different position from those granted in the United Kingdom, over which the General Council had a direct control."[53] Corrigan's motion was not carried. Even though the council ultimately approved the report, their effort did not yield a legislative result. Prospects for introducing legislation in the session rapidly dimmed as the government prioritized other more pressing matters on the University of London, prisons, and factory safety.[54]

Nearly a decade would go by before amending legislation would pass in 1886. In spite of the vagaries of parliamentary politics, the council did not lose sight of defending and expanding its authority over admission to the register.[55] But the question of opening the register to foreign and colonial medical graduates continued to be a source of insecurity within and outside of the council. In 1878 the lord president of the Privy Council the Duke of Richmond and Gordon proposed a bill in the House of Lords that included provisions dealing with compulsory conjoint examinations, the admission of women to these examinations, and the expansion of the council through elected membership. The provision for foreign and colonial medical graduates in the bill imposed steep opportunity costs. Applicants had to be at least forty years of age and legally practicing medicine in the jurisdiction where their degrees or diplomas were awarded for a minimum of ten years. The bill also extended the power of the council to register degrees and diplomas awarded in colonies and foreign countries that granted legal rights to practice to the recipients without having to sit and pass a licensing examination in the United Kingdom. It provided for separate published lists for practitioners based on the place of qualification—the United Kingdom, colonies, or foreign countries.[56]

Unable to secure passage, the lord president reintroduced his bill with amendments in the next session.[57] The bill's provision for women complicated the council's previous position. To circumvent medical authorities that refused to admit women to professional examinations, the bill provided for an additional route to the medical register, in effect a twentieth portal. The bill mandated that nonuniversity licensing bodies unite to form conjoint (medical and surgical) examinations in the three divisions of the kingdom. It also required these examinations be open to all qualified candidates—men and women. This provision was a compromise that sought to reconcile two contradictory positions: the autonomy of medical authorities and opening medicine to women.[58] The provision provided for two routes to registration within a month for those who passed the conjoint examination. First, certificate holders could apply for affiliation with a licensing body and, if approved, be registered with the corresponding title. Second, in the case of others whose application to affiliate was denied in one month's time, they could be registered on the strength of their qualifying certificate alone.

Troubled by the threat to the autonomy of medical bodies and their authority to exercise control over affiliated members, Richard Quain opposed the provisions for admitting women as well as colonial and foreign medical graduates to the register. In the event that an applicant failed to be affiliated with a licensing authority, he doubted that the council would be able to scrutinize the qualifications and character of applicants. The qualifying certificate would become a standard of entry into the register, one that would compromise public safety. This was all the more the case, Quain warned, for foreign and colonial doctors who "would be able to come to England with bogus degrees, and the Council would have to inquire (and a most onerous duty it would be) what was the value of degree at Zurich or Philadelphia; and, in short, any number of quacks or unqualified people would obtain licenses to practice without any sort of control."[59] The provision not only threatened the safety of the British public, but also was unfair to graduates when "foreigners or colonists should be able to come over to England and be placed on the Register without being examined or affiliated with a licensing body." Rather than giving the council the power to register such medical graduates, Quain proposed a motion that would grant licensing authorities the power to grant diplomas, degrees, and titles to foreign and colonial medical graduates without examination provided that they "received such evidence as to character, professional education, and examination as would be deemed sufficient as a qualification for the like degree, diplomas, or license in the case of a person not a colonial subject or a foreigner." The council would serve as a court of appeal. Quain's motion elicited divided opinion. Doubting the competency of the council to assess the qualifications of an individual without such evidence, Rolleston concurred. Simon, however, reminded members that Quain's motion contradicted the "liberal" terms for admitting colonial and foreign medical graduates that the council adopted in the wake of French legislation in 1877.[60]

Quain's resolution was carried by the committee on medical acts but faced a different outcome before the full council. Sir James Paget, who had supported the resolution as a member of the committee, reversed his opinion. Multiple portals of entry risked diluting rather than consolidating standards. "If the motion was confirmed, each authority would be at liberty to refuse to admit a foreign or colonial practitioner, and thus he might be compelled to attach himself, not to the highest authority, but to the lowest."[61] He doubted that the government would accept such a recommendation. Nor did he think it was fair to British medical graduates who sought to practice medicine outside Britain. As an alternative, Paget floated the principal of reciprocity. "Something like reciprocity should be looked for, and Englishmen should be admitted to practice in foreign countries upon somewhat the same terms as foreigners were admitted to practice here." He added that the medical corporations were no better off than the council to verify the qualifications and character of an applicant for degree or diplomas. They not only lacked standing to request information from a foreign government about diplomas or degrees, but also any information afforded by the Colonial and Foreign Office would be mediated.[62] Paget moved to withdraw Quain's proposal and prevailed.

Paget's motion returned the council to its settled consensus on the terms of the admission of foreign and colonial medical graduates to the register. A petition from the Ontario College of Physicians and Surgeons reinforced the political necessity for reciprocity. In seeking the repeal of the Medical Act, the College called for empowering colonial medical authorities to establish conditions for registering doctors in the province.[63] The reasons were a mix of the familiar and new. Alluding to the problem of the single qualification, the petition noted that a British qualification in medicine, surgery, or midwifery did not necessarily guarantee competence in all branches of medicine. Nor was the training that British graduates received necessarily appropriate for Canada: "A number of diseases are necessarily treated differently in Canada and the United Kingdom on account for the differences, climatic and physical; so that, in the interests of the public it is necessary for medical students and professional men to receive a practical medical education in Canada, or undergo an examination as to the fitness to deal with such distinctive diseases." Quite apart from the threat to public safety, the privileges called into question Britain's relations with self-governing colonies. "The Imperial legislation referred to is practically in opposition to the spirit of the British North America Act, which assumed to please the people of Ontario to deal with their civil rights."[64] The Privy Council of Canada amplified the petitioners' argument, stating "It is obvious that if this legislation is made permissible with respect to the medical profession, it might with equal propriety be extended by the Imperial Parliament to every profession, trade, and occupation in Canada, and would thus be subversive of the rights of self-government graciously conceded to the people of the Dominion."[65]

Because of the political gravity of the situation, the Privy Council sought the views of the council. Mr. Jenkyns, legal counsel for the council, acknowledged the 1858 Medical Act was designed to protect British doctors. "To preserve the rights conferred by the Medical Act of 1858, it was necessary to provide that if the colonial legislature itself requires such registration it shall not take away those rights, and shall be bound to register such a practitioner without further examination." But he did not regard the current bill as jeopardizing these rights. On the contrary, reciprocity guarantees the rights of registered doctors while acknowledging the autonomy of self-governing territories. Jenkyns asserted that "the interests of Canada would appear to be to maintain the privileges given by the Act of 1858, as, if the pending Bill passes, a holder of an Ontario diploma will be registered in the United Kingdom Register, and thus be able to practice under his Canadian diploma throughout Her Majesty's dominions."[66]

Jenkyns was not alone in endorsing the bill. The law officer of the Privy Council was even more explicit in emphasizing that the bill comported with the intent of the British North America Act.

> Although we cannot admit any limitation to the constitutional power of the Imperial Parliament to pass laws extending to the Dominion of Canada as well as other parts of Her Majesty's Dominion: we think it was intended by the British North America Act to leave such matters as the regulations for Medical and Dental Practitioners to be dealt with by the Provinces of the Canadian Dominion. We are therefore of opinion that the maintenance of those Imperial Acts which in these respects restrict the power of the Provincial Legislatures in enacting the British North America Act and that such Acts so far as they affect Canada should be repealed.[67]

Privy Council officials soon began drafting reciprocity clauses for the larger government bill to amend the Medical Act. Underlying the clauses to repeal the sections of the existing act and to grant colonial legislatures the power to reciprocate with Britain was a practical goal: ensuring that British doctors continued to enjoy unrestricted access to medical markets in exchange for admitting overseas doctors to the medical register. Little came of these efforts. Although the lord president's bill passed a second reading in the lower house, the government appointed a select committee to consider several bills to amend the Medical Act. With the collapse of the Conservative government in 1879, all legislative action was halted.

Given the manifest and persistent interests in medical education and licensing, the liberal government appointed a royal commission in 1882. As a body charged with evaluating the working of the Medical Act and receiving evidence and testimony, the commission's recommendations would provide a starting point for compromise legislation on a range of matters that continued to roil the profession, including the discretion of the GMC to admit overseas medical graduates to the register. But as the commission heard evidence, opening the register to overseas-trained doctors became linked with other issues such as a mandatory conjoint examination.

The GMC had long argued for conjoint examinations. Under the 1858 Medical Act, practitioners were entitled to be admitted to the register on the strength of a single qualification in medicine, surgery, or midwifery. The council was confident that a conjoint examination would introduce greater uniformity in training and better equip future practitioners by testing for a wider range of competencies. Opponents viewed the proposed examination as an unwarranted extension of the power of the GMC, one that subjected domestic medical graduates to a double standard.[68] They were required to pass the proposed examination to be admitted to the register while overseas-trained doctors were not. Instead, the council would determine whether they were fit to practice medicine in the United Kingdom. Cambridge

University professor of anatomy Sir George Murray Humphry, who was a former president of the local British Medical Association, was sharply critical of the double standard. "If we distrust the examining bodies in the United Kingdom, over whom we have control and whose examinations we can test, so far as to require the members who pass those examinations to pass further examination of a conjoint board, then I think that all foreigners who have passed examinations, of which we really have not much knowledge, and over which we can exercise no control, should also be required to pass such an examination."[69]

The commission chair, the Earl of Camperdon, pressed council president Paget to justify waiving the requirement for a single national examination for colonial graduates. "A man brings a diploma of the University of Madras, and you are satisfied that it is a good university, and you register him, and allow him to practice. The next day a man brings you a diploma showing that he has a first class degree and you will not allow him to practice?" He added "Does it not appear to you extraordinary that a proposal should be made that a foreign or colonial university known to be inferior to our universities, or that the majority of them, shall have its diplomas recognized so as to entitle the holder of it to practice in this country without examination." Paget's assurance of the "constant and careful supervision of the Medical Council" was no guarantee against practitioners who came from "not only the United States, but great colonies of England with English-speaking people, and very often English born people, who might come over and practice in this country, not in inconsiderable numbers, if they had advantage over our native-born subjects." Paget invoked the ties of nation and culture to reconcile the application of a double standard. "It was felt that with regard to them that they were practically Englishmen." Camperdon queried, "Why should a man taking his degree in Melbourne and who, you say, is practically, an Englishman, have an advantage over a man taking a degree in the University of Edinburgh, who I will assume to be actually an Englishman?" Paget could only reply that "when the Englishman, who has been educated and examined after the English fashion, comes here, it seems hard to say 'you shall be examined."[70]

After nearly three decades, Parliament adopted a major overhaul of the 1858 Medical Act in 1886. The Medical Amendment Act largely reinforced the jurisdiction of British medicine. The act mandated conjoint examination among nonuniversity licensing bodies and required candidates for admission to be qualified in two of three areas, namely medicine, surgery, or midwifery. The provision for reciprocity in part 2 created a new route to the register for overseas-trained doctors. But admission was not necessarily automatic. The political leadership of territories in the empire and countries had to agree to undertake to treat British doctors equitably as a condition of reciprocity. The act also empowered the GMC to determine whether medical graduates from reciprocating territories or countries were fit to practice medicine. The standard was whether medical qualifications obtained overseas afforded a "sufficient guarantee of the possession of the requisite knowledge and skill for the efficient practice of medicine, surgery and midwifery" in the United Kingdom. Although provision was made for successful candidates to be placed on the register, they were listed in a separate section for colonial and foreign doctors. Other features of the act were designed to protect or at least minimize competition from overseas-trained doctors in the domestic medical market. Residential requirements stipulated that all British-born applicants with colonial degrees had to have resided outside the United Kingdom for at least five years and those born in the colonies had to have obtained their degree while not resident in the United Kingdom.[71]

Conclusion

Both the territorial and social boundaries of British medicine privileged white, male medical graduates of university and nonuniversity medical bodies in the United Kingdom. The GMC facilitated this relationship both passively and actively. The eligibility conditions for imperial service did not fall under the control of the council. But the requirement that all candidates possess qualification from one of the nineteen licensing bodies in the United Kingdom allied British medicine with the defense and expansion of Britain's territorial empire. This requirement greatly limited the number of nonwhite colonial subjects who could realistically qualify and join the imperial services, thus defining the racial makeup of British medicine as white and male. To the extent that it could, the GMC policed the jurisdiction of British medicine. Until 1876 the council opposed any change that minimized access to unrestricted practice within the empire to registered British-educated doctors or opened it to foreign and colonial medical graduates. This position simultaneously protected the imperial market exclusively for British male medical graduates and preserved the gendered configuration of national medicine. Legislative changes in 1868 (which empowered local or colonial authorities to control access to their markets) and 1876, which (which empowered licensing bodies to permit women to sit for examinations) did not alter the essential character of British medicine. It was an imperial profession where any white male registered doctor could practice medicine wherever the union jack flew.

The council's position evolved on opening the register to foreign and colonial medical graduates. It embraced the relaxation of conditions for admission to the register to the extent that its power was expanded to recognize foreign and colonial qualifications that provided a "sufficient guarantee of the efficient practice of medicine, surgery, and medicine." This became a practical necessity when host countries, such as France and later Italy, required foreign medical graduates (i.e., British doctors) to requalify as a condition to practice. The extension of mutual reciprocal rights to practice, subject to the council's recognition, provided a compromise. Reciprocity promised a form of regulated access to the medical market of the United Kingdom and empire while ensuring the right of British doctors to practice in participating colonial possessions and foreign countries. To be sure, reciprocity enabled the council to manage the boundaries of British medicine in the world. It did not necessarily mitigate the tensions between Britain and its colonies and foreign countries. Before and after World War I, local and colonial interests clashed with national and imperial interests over the rights of doctors on the register with third country qualifications to access the medical markets of all countries and territories with whom Britain reciprocated.

Chapter Two

Expanding the Boundaries of British Medicine to Foreign and Colonial Doctors, 1886–1919

Introduction

The 1886 Medical Amendment Act reinforced the political nature of British medicine. The extension of reciprocity made possible through part 2 of the 1886 Act provided Britain with a mechanism to protect and project its interests in the world, including securing the right to practice abroad for British registered doctors, ensuring access to British medical services for the well-being of tourists and health restoration of the chronically ill living or traveling abroad, and building and sustaining strategic partnerships with territories inside and countries outside the empire.

Yet for all of the benefits associated with reciprocity, the expansion of the jurisdiction of British medicine was not without tension or conflict between the GMC and the state. Reconciling state interests in the world within the framework of the medical register, whose purpose was to serve the public by privileging British doctors, did not always align due to the uneven division of responsibility concerning the jurisdiction of British medicine. The government extended reciprocity as an act of state, and the GMC recognized the medical degrees awarded in a participating territory or country for purposes of admission to the register. Concerns about opening the domestic market to overseas-trained doctors as well as the equitable treatment of British doctors in reciprocating countries surfaced in deliberations and consultations about extending reciprocity. At the same time, enforcing the rights of doctors on the register to the unrestricted practice within the jurisdiction of British medicine was a constant preoccupation of the council. While the reciprocity agreements that Britain entered into created one of the largest medical markets in the world, participating colonial professions attempted to protect their local markets from the resulting competition by mandating conditions that either privileged local graduates or doctors who qualified or worked in the United Kingdom exclusively.

As I will show in this chapter, these reciprocating relationships proved to be critical to Britain during World War I. By the 1890s, the trend in new domestic admissions to the register settled into a fairly reliable annual average of 1,200. This number replaced total departures due to death or retirement, leaving a slight surplus of 300. The relatively tight supply of doctors contributed to the improved economic rewards of medicine before the outbreak of war in 1914. But as the war lengthened to a struggle of attrition, the personnel needs of the British military rapidly exhausted the surplus of doctors. Meeting the needs of the military without jeopardizing the civilian population became a source of continuing tension between the medical profession and the British government. The foreign and colonial list of the medical register proved to be a valuable resource. Recruiting doctors from reciprocating countries and territories as well as extending reciprocity to others relieved some of the pressure on the domestic medical profession. There was another benefit to opening the register during this period of wartime. The admission of overseas-trained doctors from foreign and Commonwealth countries served wartime propaganda goals. Their participation displayed the political scope of support of the war effort and Britain's leadership. Together, these benefits largely outweighed what was seen in Britain as the chief potential liability of reciprocity, namely a sharp increase in overseas doctors who were now eligible to practice medicine in the United Kingdom. This drawback did not become a reality. Most of the foreign-trained doctors that registered because of the war effort did so to defend the mother country or, in the case of displaced Belgian doctors, to continue to practice medicine during the German occupation of their country. The importance of family ties and access to social networks to career success undoubtedly advantaged domestic graduates and, simultaneously, checked resettlement in Britain by foreign graduates.

Reciprocating Countries on the Foreign List

Reciprocity did not lead to overseas doctors swamping the domestic medical market. Britain only entered into reciprocal arrangements with two countries: Italy in 1901 and Japan in 1905 (see table 2.1). The number of practitioners who were admitted to the foreign list was modest. Of the forty-three doctors who were admitted two were from Japan and forty-one were from Italy.[1]

It is likely that the very mechanism for promoting the movement of doctors across borders actually inhibited its implementation on a wider scale. Reciprocity involved a political decision that few countries were prepared

Table 2.1. Reciprocating territories in the British Empire and foreign countries, 1886–1914

Foreign countries	British territories
Italy	Ceylon
Japan	Hong Kong
Belgium	India
	Malta
	New Zealand
	Newfoundland
	Straits Settlement (Singapore, Malacca, Dingding, and Penang)
	Australia (New South Wales, South Australia, and Victoria)
	Canada (Manitoba, New Brunswick, Nova Scotia, Ontario, Prince Edward Island, Quebec, North-West Territories, Alberta, and Saskatchewan)

Source: "Medical Register" (London: General Medical Council, 1920), ixxxiii.

to undertake. Until the passage of the 1886 Medical Act, Britain was not alone in guarding access to its market to order to protect members of its national profession from competition. Requalification, as opposed to recognizing foreign medical qualifications, was common throughout Europe. In general, foreign doctors seeking to practice medicine legally had to obtain a qualification in the host country. This involved sitting and passing a state examination and sometimes also obtaining a new university degree. Some countries were more demanding than others. For example, in Austria, "naturalization as an Austrian subject" was a "necessary preliminary" to enrolling in the university. The examination in Belgium was a barrier to practice for foreigners. "So stringent are the formalities that it is held by His Majesty's Minister at Brussels that the difficulties are prohibitive. No foreigner has, as a matter of fact, received permission to practice since 1893."[2]

Italy, 1900–1905

Compared to other continental markets, Italy was open to British practitioners. Nearly one hundred British doctors established practices in Italy to serve the needs of the British nationals who visited Italian health spas and other tourist destinations. Under the Public Health Act of 1888, foreign practitioners were permitted to practice among British residents in the country without special permission. Unrestricted private practice, by contrast, required the permission of one of seven Royal Universities that acted in the name of the Italian state. But Italy's relative openness to British doctors did not last.

Italian doctors—much like French doctors—sought to limit access to the medical market. Through local medical boards or *Ordine dei Medici,* they lobbied the Minister of Public Instruction.[3] Under proposed legislation in 1890, British doctors would be required to requalify in Italy by obtaining a university degree in medicine. J. J. Eyre of Rome appealed to the GMC for assistance. Although the council lacked standing to officially intervene, council president Richard Quain forwarded Eyre's letter to the Privy Council.[4] In his letter to the lord president, Quain described the proposed legislation as little more than "protection" for Italian doctors. He contrasted the intentions of the legislation with the privileges foreign doctors enjoyed in Britain, though he conveniently omitted mentioning their disqualification from the rights of practice to which registered doctors were entitled. Alluding to the hurdles to practice in Europe more generally, Quain warned that the proposed legislation if enacted would be "unjust" to British practitioners and "highly injurious to the many subjects of Her Majesty who travel for recreation in foreign countries, or frequent foreign health resorts, which in a large proportion of cases owe their prosperity almost wholly to British practitioners who have settled there."[5] Quain urged the government to go on the offensive. To strengthen Britain's negotiating hand, he proposed amending legislation that would prohibit unregistered foreign doctors from the privilege of practice.[6]

Meanwhile, Count F. De Renzis, the Italian ambassador to Britain, approached Foreign Secretary the Marquis of Salisbury about whether or not Italian doctors could practice in Britain without obtaining further qualifications and, if not, whether the government would grant permission to practice to Italian nationals only.[7] Through the Privy Council, the Foreign Office solicited the views of the GMC. The council conveyed mixed messages. Initially, the executive committee welcomed "such recognition of a right by English practitioners to practice in Italy, as would enable Her Majesty in Council, under section XVII of Part II of the Medical Act, 1886, to extend similar privileges to Italian practitioners in this country."[8] But the council was not unanimous in its support of this position. Some members regarded the executive committee's response to the Privy Council as overly hasty, committing the council to a policy that was by no means settled or for that matter legally possible. Though the number of Italian doctors who were to benefit from such a policy was small, several members strongly opposed extending recognition. Dr. McVail warned of a double standard in the admission to the register. "Why should the council compel Englishmen, Irishmen, and Scotsmen to undergo a very difficult examination and yet allow foreign practitioners to practice in this country without inquiring what training they had had?" Fearing that the domestic profession would be "swamped by foreign immigrants," Victor Horsley, who was the first directly elected member to the council, preferred to privilege reciprocity within the empire, "whose people were our own relations, and who could converse in our own language." Horsley added that as a directly elected representative of the profession, he believed that the council should act in the interest of the public as well as the medical profession.[9]

The council sought legal counsel regarding the legality of restricting the rights of foreign-trained doctors on the register. M. Muir MacKenzie scrutinized the sections of the Medical Act that related to reciprocity with foreign countries. Admission to the register for foreign medical graduates was a two-stage process, related both to the foreign graduate's country of origin and the graduate's medical qualifications. First, under section 17 of the Medical Act, the Privy Council could only extend such privileges if registered British doctors in the foreign country were afforded "such privileges of practicing in the foreign country as to Her Majesty may seem just." Second, under section 12 of the Medical Act, the council had to be satisfied that the applicant's qualification was equivalent to British medical education and training. Once admitted to the register, foreign medical graduates were entitled to the unrestricted practice of medicine. According to Mackenzie, "there is no expressed provision . . . which empowers Her Majesty, by Order in Council which applies to the Act to a foreign state, to limit the right of the foreign practitioners, by virtue of the order in Council and the Act, being entitled to be registered."[10]

This opinion reflected the political logic underlying the continuing debates over the jurisdiction of British medicine. For licensing and nonlicensing bodies, anything that smacked of differential treatment would have doomed political support for a national body that regulated and controlled the profession in the United Kingdom. The benefits—which were many—and the responsibilities—which were few—of admission to the register associated doctors with British medicine regardless of where they obtained their qualifications. The need to codify the privileges of British practitioners in foreign countries reinforced the principle of equitable treatment for all admitted to the register whether qualified in the United Kingdom or not. But the legal interpretation of the 1886 Medical Act emphasized the disparity between the underlying assumption of professional equity extended to foreign doctors on the British medical register and the differential treatment of British doctors contemplated in Italy. Adopting a more politically ambiguous position, the executive committee presented MacKenzie's letter by indicating "difficulties that surround the granting of recognition of medical graduates over whose curriculum of study in professional examinations the General Medical Council can exercise no supervision."

Although the term *difficulties* was vague, its implication was clear enough: Italian qualifications were suspect. But Stuart Tidney, a longtime resident of Italy, disputed this implication in a letter to the *British Medical Journal* (*BMJ*): "It should be borne in mind that we alone of the more advanced European States have a number of licensing corporations varying in the severity of their examination tests, while each member of the more important Continental States has the 'one-portal' system." He warned that putting off an agreement with Italy for too long was likely to jeopardize a relationship with the one country where British doctors were received "courteously."[11] If there was any remaining doubt about accepting the unequal conditions under which British doctors would be expected to practice, a joint letter from British nationals in Italy to Lord Currie, the British representative in Rome, clarified their position. Edmonston Charles, John J. Eyre, and G. Sandison Brock urged extending reciprocity as proposed by the Italian government.[12]

In early 1900, the lord president activated part 2 of the Medical Act. Satisfied that privileges were "just" for British doctors, the Privy Council extended reciprocal privileges to those Italian doctors who were admitted to the register after the council was satisfied of their fitness to practice medicine. In arriving at its decision, the Privy Council gave primary consideration to the existing and future health needs of British nationals living or traveling in Italy. Predictably, the GMC objected to extending reciprocity.[13] Horsley moved a resolution: "That the Council would urge Her Majesty's Government to use its influence with the Italian Government in promoting legislation on this subject so as to ensure for English practitioners such full privilege of practice in Italy as would be conceded by the law of this country."[14] George Brown echoed Horsley, asking "if the General Medical Council was to stand by and do nothing whilst the privileges of English practitioners were being batted away?" For Cambridge University member Donald MacAlister, such a representation carried risks of antagonizing the Privy Council. Still others regarded the "see fit" power of the medical council as more properly within its competency than the political extension of reciprocal privileges. Sir Dyce Duckworth reminded his colleagues that "the council had the absolute power of saying who should come here and practice, because in order to be registered the applicant must satisfy the council as to character, education, and so on." In light of Duckworth's observation, the adoption of Horsley's resolution allowed the council to register its views without sacrificing their power to control access to the register.[15] While the council objected to the decision of the Privy Council, its worries did not bear fruit. Before the outbreak of World War I, only forty-one Italian nationals had registered since 1901.[16] The terms of reciprocity were also modified to equalize the conditions of practice for British practitioners. A 1910 decree removed this disparity and permitted doctors on the register to practice among nationals as well as nonnationals in Italy.[17]

Japan, 1905–16

Where the politics of reciprocity with Italy reflected the priority assigned to the interests of British nationals, the decision to extend reciprocity to Japan in 1906 was largely driven by the promotion of Anglo-Japanese relations.[18] Until the mid-nineteenth century, Japan's interaction with western powers was limited. The impact of US-led gunboat diplomacy beginning in 1853–54 and the collapse of the *shogunate* order laid the foundation for the intensification of diplomacy, trade and commerce, and education and cultural exchanges. These contacts and others spurred the modernization of society and the state in Japan. Western medicine formed part of this landscape of change. By 1900 medical education—based on the German model—was established at the two principal Imperial Universities at Tokyo (1886) and Kyoto (1897). The university bachelor and medical degrees (*Igakuhakushi* and *Igakushi*) were supplemented by medical diplomas awarded by *igaku semmon gakko* or technical colleges. These colleges were sponsored by government jurisdictions (prefecture and municipality) as well as private entities.[19] Furthermore, Japan adopted licensing regulations that specifically made provisions for foreign doctors to practice in Japan subject to the permission of the minister of the interior.[20]

By the turn of the twentieth century, Japan had emerged as a major power and exerted influence in East Asia, especially the Korean Peninsula, while harboring ambitions for mainland China and Southeast Asia. Its resounding defeat of Russia in 1905 announced Japan's arrival on the world stage. In order to promote stability in the Pacific and to preserve British influence in the region, the United Kingdom entered into an agreement with Japan in 1902 and renewed it in 1905, and again in 1911. For its part, this agreement facilitated Japan's economic activity in the region via the British territorial empire in the Straits Settlements and Malaya. In these territories, Japan had established an economic footprint primarily consisting of farming and extraction industries for domestic consumption and reexport.

In fact, the occasion for the 1905 request for the application of part 2 of the Medical Act to Japan was the adoption of a local ordinance regulating the registration of practitioners in the British Straits Settlement. The ordinance made the registration of practitioners conditional on the possession of "a degree or license in medicine and surgery of any medical school in the Empire of Japan" recognized by the GMC for admission to the foreign list of the medical register in the United Kingdom.[21] In asking the Foreign Office to facilitate the application of the Medical Act to Japan, the representative of the Japanese Legation, Tadasu Hayashi, based his request on a combination of professional equity and the parity of medical training in Japan with that of the West.

> In view of the fact that Japan has long since been granting, without examination, the license for practicing medicine to any British medical practitioners who possess recognized British diplomas or who are duly registered in the *Medical Register* of the United Kingdom, and also of the fact that the ability and knowledge of the Japanese medical practitioners amply entitle them to be registered as such in any art of the United Kingdom, the Imperial Government earnestly hopes that the British Government will see their way to cause some measures to be taken by which Japan shall be recognized as one of the countries to which the Medical Act applies.[22]

While the Foreign Office solicited the assistance of the council, it explored the possibility of a more immediate accommodation via the Colonial Office to enable Japanese doctors to practice in British colonies. This accommodation involved amending the local ordinance "so as to exclude the condition in regards the recognition of Japanese Degrees, Diplomas, and Licenses in the United Kingdom."[23]

The council requested and received additional information regarding the conditions for medical licenses granted by the Japanese minister of the interior. These included two routes: those who passed the state general medical examination and medical graduates of the Imperial Universities and *igaku semmon gakko*, or technical colleges. Hayashi drew attention to the rigor of the education and training: "I may point out that before students enter Medical College they must finish the course of Grammar School, Middle School, and Preparatory School for the university, which extends over at least 14 years in all." He added in reference to the nonuniversity schools that "the qualification of the candidate and subjects of lessons are nearly the same as in the University, the course extending over four years."[24] Writing to the Privy Council in anticipation of the GMC's decision, registrar H. E. Allen lowered expectations in terms of the qualifications likely to be recognized. "If the precedents of India and Italy are followed, the Council's recognition would probably be limited to the Medical Degrees granted by the Imperial University of Japan." This preference would certainly ensure a fair degree of harmonization and reflect the Council's relative lack of familiarity with the nonuniversity medical schools. At the same time, the preference for university medical degrees would also reinforce a distinction among practitioners of western medicine in Japan, including the unrestricted right to practice in the British Empire.[25] The council recommended the application of the Medical Act to Japan.

In the meantime, the executive committee deferred consideration of the recognition of nonuniversity diplomas until 1914. In the interim, the changes adopted ranged from standardizing the curriculum based on the bachelor of medicine degree, regulating the final professional examinations, and providing oversight of medical education and registration.[26] The responsiveness of Japan to these conditions reflected an ongoing commitment to modernizing its institutions and to securing the recognition of western powers as a peer. Indeed, this period coincided with changes to the Anglo-Japan Agreement. Originally renewed in 1905, the agreement was renewed twice more in 1908 and 1911. The terms broadened cooperation between the empires. In exchange for the recognition of British interests in the region, the United Kingdom validated Japan's hegemony over Korea and facilitated its entry into Britain's territories in the Pacific such as Australia. Reciprocity continued to serve these essentially political purposes. After consolidating its control over Korea, Japan extended its law regulating the practice of medicine to the Korean Peninsula, including the unrestricted rights of British registered practitioners on the medical register to practice.[27]

In 1914 Japan raised the matter of recognition of nonuniversity medical diplomas. Leading this effort was the Central Sanitary Council of Japan. Chaired by the surgeon-general and member of the house of peers Baron Tadanori Ishiguro, the membership of the council comprised graduates of the Imperial universities, members of the national academy, and senior government officials.[28] Kitasato Shibasaburo stood out. A student at the University of Berlin (1885–91) under the direction of one of Europe's leading bacteriologists, Robert Koch, Shibasaburo was renowned for his contributions to the field, which led to his election to the British Royal Society and the honorary title of professor of the German Empire.[29] For the Central Sanitary Council, the continued delay in Britain's recognition of nonuniversity medical degrees did more than threaten professional relations between the two empires; it also imperiled the health of nationals living in British Straits Settlements and Federated Malay States who were denied access to Japanese practitioners. They warned that the status quo "will in the end prove deleterious to the commercial relations between the two countries."[30]

The Central Sanitary Council's letter was submitted to the Foreign Office by the Japanese ambassador as part of an official request from the government of Japan. In forwarding the request to the medical council via the Privy Council, the Colonial Office conveyed its willingness to accommodate Japan. "It is urgently desired that a settlement of this long-standing question may be reached without delay," the under secretary of state wrote on behalf of Colonial Secretary Bonar Law.[31] In the meantime, Law sought the approval of the medical council to amend the local ordinance to permit medical graduates of nonuniversity medical colleges to practice in British territories.[32] After reviewing Japan's changes to the Medical School curriculum, plans for a final professional examination, and the general regulation of the register in Japan, A. J. Cockington forwarded the dossier to council president MacAlister for approval, which was granted.[33]

Ensuring that nationals had access to registered doctors or promoting political relations with imperial Japan led the Privy Council to apply part 2 of the Medical Act to the Kingdom of Italy and the Empire of Japan respectively. Reciprocity did not necessarily mean equality for British doctors in Italy. Seeking to preserve their practices, they requested narrowly tailored rights to practice only among British nationals even though Italian doctors would have unrestricted rights to the British medical market. Even though the council objected, it had neither the power nor authority to reverse the decision of the Privy Council. Where the council did exercise authority was over the recognition of the medical qualifications of participating countries. As in the case of Japan, the approval of the GMC effectively reproduced British medicine as a universal, or at least a western, norm of medicine. At the same time, the very conditional nature of recognition invested in the council the power to determine whether a country or territory conformed to a constructed category of national medicine.

Reciprocating Territories in the Empire: The Colonial List

The application of part 2 of the Medical Act to the territories of the British Empire was far more common than to foreign countries. Between 1887 and 1914, New Zealand, India, and several states and provinces in the federated dominions of Australia and Canada gained reciprocity with the United Kingdom (see table 5). The GMC recognized the medical qualifications of twelve universities and four medical colleges or professional bodies.

While registration for participating territories was a new departure, it was built on conforming to standards already established by the council. One of the council's early achievements in upgrading medical training involved the adoption of minimum eligibility requirements to sit for the final professional examinations administered by university and nonuniversity licensing bodies in the United Kingdom. All applicants were required to present evidence of having completed a university general education or its equivalent—such as a diploma, degree, or an examination certificate—before either commencing or, at least, completing four years of mandatory medical training.

Each year the GMC published in the medical press an annual list of approved diplomas, degrees, and certificates that individual university and nonuniversity licensing bodies would accept from colonial and foreign institutions. The Royal College of Surgeons (England) recognized colonial degrees and certificates from the universities of Calcutta, Madras, and Bombay in India; McGill in Montreal, Queen's College, Kingston, and Victoria College, Toronto, in Canada; Codrington College in Barbados; and

Tasmanian Council of Education in colonial Australia. The Royal Colleges of Physicians and Surgeons in Edinburgh made similar provision to accept degrees from colonial and foreign universities and colleges, as did the universities of Edinburgh, Glasgow, Aberdeen, and St. Andrews. This listing was updated annually to reflect the addition of degrees and certificates adopted by individual licensing bodies or by the council at the request of colonial universities or colleges such as Christ College in New Zealand and McGill in Montreal, Canada.[34]

At the same time, the application of part 2 of the Medical Act to territories played a part in the tensions between Britain and the empire over autonomy and control. Ideally, reciprocity afforded Britain a framework for managing its empire, allowing for both a degree of autonomy in the periphery and metropolitan-led imperial unity. But aligning these goals within the jurisdiction of British medicine required constant political management on the part of the GMC. This was particularly the case when territories sought to condition or limit the scope of third country or territory reciprocity in order to protect their local markets from competition.

Malta, 1901

By 1901 Malta had been a possession of Britain for a century. Ruled by the Order of Knights Hospitaller since the sixteenth century, the island of Malta served as an outpost of the Holy Roman Empire to assist pilgrims traveling to and from the Holy Land. The order increasingly engaged in periodic armed conflicts with forces of the Ottoman Empire, culminating in the Order's successful repulse of the great siege in 1565. Later, the Napoleonic War ended the peace and security of rule by the knights. Initially seized by Napoleon while en route to Egypt, the island was liberated by Admiral Horatio Nelson, who defeated the French fleet. In 1800 Malta became part of the British Empire.

Situated in the central Mediterranean Sea, the island of Malta provided a strategic port and later coaling station for the British fleet, especially after the opening of the Suez Canal in 1869. A small British community grew up around the military and maritime installation. This community provided a market for British doctors. But rumor of negotiations between Britain and Italy raised fears of competition among local practitioners, not to mention anti-Italian sentiment.[35] Article 5 of Malta's Sanitary Ordinance was adopted to protect British doctors. It mandated one year of probationary practice in the British Isles before being registered locally. The education committee of the GMC subsequently reviewed the regulations governing the practice of medicine on the island and recommended the repeal of Article 5 of the Sanitary Ordinance.[36] This recommendation was consistent with the unrestricted nature of the rights of practice associated with registration and also removed a potential hurdle to negotiations with Italy. Malta repealed the ordinance and began reciprocating with the United Kingdom in 1901.[37]

Canada: Quebec Province

Like Malta, the provinces in the federated dominion of Canada pursued reciprocity instrumentally. Although federated in 1867, there was no dominion-wide medical body that regulated the medical profession. Instead, each province controlled access to their respective medical markets. Such autonomy certainly created economic advantages for local medical schools, colleges, and professions. Monopolies or restricted markets generally do. As Ronald Hamowy has shown, autonomy produced variable standards of education and training. Invalid beyond its jurisdiction, provincial autonomy precluded interprovincial reciprocity.[38]

These and other features of the institutional context of Canadian medicine spurred the Canadian Medical Association in 1894 to create a committee to explore the possibility of uniform educational standards while preserving the rights of provincial bodies to license doctors to practice medicine locally. Thomas Roddick, a Montreal surgeon and member of the faculty at McGill University, chaired the committee. As a Conservative member of the federal Parliament, Roddick introduced legislation for the creation of a medical council for Canada. Quite apart from promoting common standards, a dominion-wide body, he argued, would open the empire to local medical graduates.[39] Roddick's bill faced objections from provinces that feared that the authority of the new council would supplant their local bodies. The final bill, which passed in 1902, reaffirmed the power of local authorities to license. One provision of the bill, at the same time, required all provinces to enact the enabling legislation before the dominion council could be formally established.[40]

In the meantime, in 1907 Quebec initiated the process for the application of part 2 of the 1886 Medical Act. This mainly involved assuring equitable treatment for all registered doctors in the province, including those on the British register. For the most part, the council was pleased with the proposed changes in provincial legislation that achieved this larger end. But the GMC executive council raised a concern about the adoption of an ex post facto proviso by the provincial Privy Council that had been approved by the governor-general.[41]

Under the revised by-laws of the College of Physicians and Surgeons of Quebec, the right to practice medicine in the province required doctors to either obtain a certificate of admission to study medicine from the Medical Board of the Province at least four years before their admission to the medical register in the United Kingdom or to practice medicine in the United Kingdom for at least five years. MacAlister pointed out that the proviso negated the principal of equitable treatment in a letter to the lord president. "It does not appear to be included in any existing law, and the Committee are unable to understand its bearing and intention. It would seem by its terms to exclude nearly all British registered practitioners from the privilege of practicing in Quebec, as few, if any, can be expected, 'as a condition antecedent to their British registration' to have satisfied in detail 'the requirements of the Quebec medical law for the obtaining of a license to practice.' The Committee are therefore constrained to think that the terms of the proviso must have some other significance, and they suggest that you, my Lord, should make inquiry regarding it."[42] The "other significance" referred to the college's attempt to control access to its medical market. Under the conditions of reciprocity, the province would be forced to register doctors who were trained in Britain, but also those on the foreign and colonial list. Although MacAlister was far too polite to accuse the college, much less the governor-general, of seeking to circumvent the authority of the council, the insinuation was clear enough. The province ultimately modified the proviso.[43]

This was not the only occasion for tension between local and imperial interests. In 1909 the Quebec provincial legislature—at the initiative of the college—revised the language of the Quebec Medical Act. A new bylaw recently adopted by the college provided for the registration of foreign practitioners on the British medical register who had resided "outside of the Province of Quebec" for a minimum of five years. This revision to the Medical Act used the same language but substituted the phrase "in the United Kingdom." This change did not alter the right of medical graduates of the United Kingdom. It did, however, effectively prohibit foreign practitioners who were on the British register from registering in the province as a right. In a letter to the Privy Council, H. E. Allen described the implications of the new law: "The Province thus obtains the benefit of what may be described as Imperial recognition and validity for its degrees and diplomas; but it excludes from local privileges of practicing a number of 'registered medical practitioners of the United Kingdom.'" Allen objected to the unilateral action of the province: "The change has been made without any communication to the Medical Council, or, so far as is known, to the Privy Council. As it may justly be held to alter the basis on which the Order in Council was understood to be made, the Executive Committee feel bound to direct it to the notice of the Lord President."[44]

Since the revised law altered the basis for the application of the Medical Act and the recognition of the medical degrees and diplomas, the withdrawal of recognition was the only leverage that was available to the GMC. For his part, the registrar of the medical board of Quebec, J. Gauvreau, explained the revised language as a means to regulate the local profession, specifically Canadians who attempted to avoid passing the preliminary examination by obtaining a license in England and then seeking registration in Quebec. Gauvreau stressed that the law was not designed to slight the medical council, but rather to prevent "irregular physicians of our own country who refuse to comply with the requirements of our Provincial Law, to extort a license from us by way of exchange for an English one."[45] Underlying the action of the college was a desire to control interprovincial reciprocity. Without the residency requirement in the United Kingdom, the medical board of the college feared that doctors from outside of Quebec would swamp the local market.[46] Allen remained unmoved by Gauvreau's appeal to the local concerns of the Quebec profession.[47] The law was revised to the satisfaction of the council.[48]

The circumstances that led to the establishment of reciprocal relations in medicine between Britain and its territorial possessions in the empire and foreign countries were not identical. As shown in the cases of Italy and Japan, the interests of the state—accommodating the health needs of British nationals and strategic partnerships—were given priority over those of the council, which were more closely focused on equitable treatment of British doctors abroad. By contrast, the interests of the state aligned more closely with those of the council when reciprocity was considered within the empire. These cases of reciprocity built on and extended the authority of the council (representing the imperial metropole) in conferring credibility on colonial medical institutions and diplomas. The tensions associated with reciprocity within and outside of the empire underscored the very conditional nature of the alignment of local (colonial and national) interests with those of Britain. Until the outbreak of World War I, British medicine was little more than the sum of its far-flung parts. At the same time, these first steps collectively helped to define the legal foundation for the council's power to regulate doctors who were trained in one place but practiced legally in another.

World War and Political Adjustments to the Boundaries of British Medicine, 1914–19

Constraints on the capacity of university and nonuniversity bodies to produce doctors created a structural limitation on the size of the domestic profession. The 1858 Medical Act prescribed the nineteen institutions whose qualifications met the criteria for registration, a number that remained unchanged between the original act and its amendment in 1886. Parliament created six new universities in England and Wales between 1900 and 1913. All six—Birmingham (1900), Liverpool (1903), Leeds (1904), Sheffield (1905), Bristol (1909), and Wales (1911)—were entitled to hold qualifying examinations and award degrees in medicine, surgery, and midwifery for the purpose of registration. Even with the combined output of these new institutions, the size of the profession remained stable in the prewar period. On average, some 900 doctors who died or retired from practice were replaced by 1,200 new admissions to the register annually.

The reliable difference between separations and admissions to the register provided a measure of stability in the supply of doctors. Doctor-population ratios generally reflected this trend, spanning from 1/1550 (1871), 1/1700 (1881), to 1/1500 (1891). These trends coincided with others that contributed to improving economic rewards of the profession. Nationally, per capita income had doubled between 1870 and 1914 and likely translated into increased expenditures on medicine.[49] In 1911 the liberal government introduced the National Health Insurance. This government-, employer-, and employee-funded scheme, which targeted workers in highly unionized and economically volatile industries, expanded the market for medical care to include members of the working classes. As Anne Digby has shown, it provided a reliable financial safety net for panel doctors.[50] At the same time, the limited supply of doctors contributed to the persistent maldistribution of doctors in the United Kingdom, especially in underserved rural and working-class provincial communities. Furthermore, any sudden spike in the demand for doctors would be disruptive and could potentially jeopardize civilian access to medical care. The outbreak of World War I did just this.

When Britain declared war on behalf of the empire, it did so without first securing agreement of the elected governments of dominions or even consulting the dependent colonies or protectorates. Still, the threat to the mother county provided an opportunity to translate the council's new "greater empire" attitude toward British medicine into action. Reciprocity afforded all medically trained subjects of the Crown with a mechanism for answering the call to duty. Only doctors on the register were permitted to serve in the Royal Army Medical Corps (RAMC). This had been brought home during the South African War in 1901–2 for Canada's regimental personnel. Due to the lack of reciprocity between the dominion and the United Kingdom, Canadian medical personnel were prohibited from treating British wounded.[51] After that a number of provinces entered into reciprocity. Before the end of the first year of World War I, New Brunswick, Newfoundland, Ontario, and Saskatchewan provinces initiated arrangements for reciprocity. The province of British Columbia followed. A cable from the province's registrar of the College of Physicians and Surgeons of British Columbia captured the spirit of patriotism and practicality. "It has been felt for some time that in view of the present conditions, brought on largely by the war, there ought to be reciprocity between this country and Great Britain in order that there may be no question as to the standing of our men serving in Britain or on the continent."[52] In 1917 nearly 1,250 Canadian medical officers served in the RAMC in France, England, and in Canada.[53]

For Britain, reciprocity helped to underscore the political alliance arrayed against the Central Powers (Germany, the Austro-Hungarian Empire, and the Ottoman Empire). In January 1915, Belgium joined Japan and Italy to become the third foreign country to enter into a reciprocal medical agreement with Britain. A Royal Decree provided for the mutual recognition of British and Belgian qualifications during the wartime emergency.[54] Together, registered doctors from these three countries increased to 125, nearly tripling the total number since 1914. Council president MacAlister described the larger political purpose of reciprocity in his annual address: "When reciprocity is thereby arranged with South Africa, another step, and that practically the least that remains, will have been taken towards the medical confederation of the Empire. Our allies Italy, Japan, and Belgium already stand in similar relations with this country: and it may that the Council's next duty will be the endeavor to bring some form of reciprocity with other allied and friendly nations, where the standards of medical education and qualifications are not inferior to our own."[55]

Reciprocity was not simply a matter of flag-waving for Britain. It expanded its personnel capacity to deliver health care at home while engaging in a world war. Like other males swept up in the recruitment euphoria, medical students and practitioners were optimistic that the war, begun in the late summer of 1914, would be over by Christmas. Beyond the exemption for fourth- and fifth-year medical students and the minimum age eligibility of eighteen, there were no limitations for young men interested in joining the military. In light of the replacement trend in the supply of doctors, changes in the number of medical students directly impacted the supply and characteristics of future doctors. As table 6 shows, the projected yield of graduates in 1917 and 1918—based on second- and third-year students in 1911 and 1912—totaled 2,285. By contrast, the yield for 1919 and 1920 students, based on 1912 and 1913 enrollments, was 1,760. The 525 (29 percent) difference put the 1919 and 1920 yields below prewar replacement numbers. The gender characteristics of medical student were not unaffected. In fact, from 1911 to 1915, the percentage of male medical students declined from a prewar high of 87 percent to 69 percent, while female students experienced an unprecedented increase from 13 percent to 31 percent (see table 2.2). These trends were disquieting to the Central Medical War Committee. Frederick Taylor, the president of the Royal College of Physicians and chairman of the committee, argued that increasing the number of women was neither a short- nor long-term solution for military and civilian needs: "It should be pointed out that they are not suitable for all hospital appointments nor for all forms of general practice, and of course are not available for the Navy and Army. It must therefore not be assumed that an increase on women doctors can compensate for a serious shortage of male doctors."[56]

Table 2.2. Entrants to medical school and projections of future medical graduates, 1911–21

Entered as students in					
1915	in 1916	Men	Women	Total	Eligible to qualify in
1915	1st Year	1422	636	2056	1921
1914	2nd Year	783	295	1078	1920
1913	3rd Year	519	163	682	1919
1912	4th Year	1078	145	1223	1918
1911	5th Year	922	140	1062	1917

Source: Frederick Taylor, Central War Committee Memorandum on Shortage of Medical Students, August 30, 1917, NATS 1/814, pp. 1–2.

According to Edwin Cornwall, the minister of National Health Insurance, the supply of domestic registered practitioners was under strain as well.[57] The lack of stability in the number of medical students was mirrored in the profession. From the turn of the twentieth century through the first year of the war, the total number of doctors in Britain ranged from a low of 36,000 to a high of 43,000, or between 1 doctor per 666 people and 1 per 558 respectively. But these ratios became even less favorable when the state adjusted the age of military eligibility and reduced the medical school exemptions. Of the nearly 30,000 registered doctors in 1917, some 13,284 directly or indirectly supported an army of five million while the remaining 14,718 served the civilian population of twenty-four million. This shift of practitioners from civilian to state service yielded decidedly unfavorable ratios: now there was only one doctor per 2,344 persons in the civilian population and one doctor per 376 military personnel. As Britain prepared for a major offense on the western front and in the eastern Mediterranean, the call for another four hundred practitioners to serve led all medical advisory bodies, including the Central Medical War Committee, the Royal Colleges of Physicians and Surgeons, and the Medical Students and Schools Committee, to object to this requisition, lest civilian health be irreversibly compromised. It was an indication of how grave the situation had become when the government adopted in the Man-Power Act in 1918. This act subjected all males from eighteen to fifty-five, unless exempted, to conscription. The age eligibility was specifically extended to fifty-five for doctors.[58]

In light of the strain on Britain's medical personnel, reciprocity was advantageous for increasing the supply of doctors. As cohort sizes shrunk in medical schools, colonial and foreign practitioners enabled Britain to maintain its overall average production of new admissions to the medical register. Its five-year (1915–19) average of 1,252 was slightly higher than for the period between 1896 and 1919. Before 1914 the combined colonial and foreign lists averaged 4 percent to 5 percent of all new admissions. After 1914 their proportion never fell below 10 percent and peaked at 34 percent in 1919 (see table 2.3). The combined wartime totals ranged from an equivalent to a full and quarter size of a medical school.

Table 2.3. Annual admissions to the British Medical Register for England, Scotland, and Ireland, and foreign and colonial medical graduates, 1896–1919

Year	England	Scotland	Ireland	Colonial	Foreign	Total
1896	774	477	128	6	—	1385
1897	662	425	135	8	—	1230
1898	611	460	131	8	—	1210
1899	696	487	156	12	—	1351
1900	669	499	170	7	—	1345
1901	653	499	147	18	1	1318
1902	654	432	158	27	4	1275
1903	658	435	126	10	4	1233
1904	612	388	156	9	3	1168
1905	620	450	138	28	4	1240
1906	596	415	170	13	3	1197
1907	563	466	170	18	4	1221
1908	536	408	165	24	4	1137
1909	504	435	157	43	4	1143
1910	444	397	171	45	5	1062
1911	484	339	173	38	8	1042
1912	540	376	188	52	1	1157
1913	528	365	210	61	4	1168
1914	666	445	245	76	1	1433
1915	594	412	251	181	88	1526
1916	542	344	186	123	7	1202
1917	494	321	172	141	8	1134
1918	429	289	195	148	16	1077
1919	378	284	210	436	14	1322
Average for 1898–1919						1232
Average for 1915–19						1252

Source: Table E from the "Medical Register" (London: General Medical Council, 1920), ixxvii.

If anything, the entry of the United States into the war in late 1917 only highlighted the importance of the tactical reserve of reciprocating countries and territories. "The welcome cooperation of the United States of America, in sending over medical units in advance of its troops, has afforded the allies some relief in that respect," MacAlister observed in his presidential address in the fall of 1917.[59] But it proved to be only a temporary benefit. "Officers of the American Medical Service have accepted honorary or other temporary positions in hospitals at home and abroad, and have thus released British officers and practitioners for other work. But we shall not be able to count on this help after the arrival in Europe of the American forces in full strength." Nor was American civilian labor accessible. "And, again, we cannot count on American civilian practitioners to furnish many accessions to our Register. In the absence of Federal legislation authorizing professional reciprocity between the United States and Britain, His Majesty is debarred from applying the Medical Act, 1886, to American medical practitioners to the Register unless they pass a recognized examination in medicine, surgery and midwifery, and so acquire a professional title registerable in this country." In the meantime, MacAlister reminded his audience that the council had maximized reciprocity to the full extent possible. "Where such legislation, within or without the Empire, has already been accomplished, the Council has not failed to give it effect. Already the Foreign and Colonial List of the Register include over 1,000 practitioners, and their legal status in regard is the same as our own."[60]

Conclusion

By the end of the war, the boundaries of British medicine in the world were more unified than at any other time. Belgium joined Japan and Italy among reciprocating foreign countries. Five more provinces in the largest North American dominion increased the total Canadian number to nine. The annual number of admissions to the foreign and colonial list increased three and five times respectively between 1896 and 1919. The addition of foreign-trained service personnel supplemented Britain's critically low domestic supply of medical personnel. These benefits were scarcely imagined in 1886 when reciprocity became a formal mechanism for monitoring the rights of doctors within the territorial boundaries of British medicine. On the contrary, the council was decidedly unenthusiastic about extending reciprocity to Italy, much less Japan. In both cases, the interests of the council were subordinated to the priorities of the state. Even the process of managing relations with reciprocating territories in the empire proved to be fraught with tension over local control of access to colonial medical markets and the entitlement of any doctors on the register to practice legally in any territory that reciprocated with Britain.

Yet this period created the conditions for transforming the register into a global medium of British medicine. In defining the rights of all doctors on the register, the council endowed admission to the register with the principal of equality. In the context of a global war, the register functioned as a tool to mobilize the world on behalf of Britain. For existing and new countries and colonies that reciprocated with Britain, admission to the register had the benefit of enhancing the supply of their medical personnel. It not only permitted registered doctors to treat British military personnel and serve in British units, but also helped to ensure that the civilian population across the empire was not denied access to British medical graduates. The political symbolism of reciprocity was no less potent. It enabled Britain to harness the labor of doctors trained outside of the United Kingdom on its own terms while underscoring international and Commonwealth support for its wartime leadership.

Chapter Three

Autonomy and Control

Managing British Medicine in the Age of Decolonization, 1919–30

Introduction

Shortly after the return to peacetime in 1919, challenges to the reach of British medicine emerged that would persist throughout the interwar period. The national and imperial boundaries that had opened the world to British medicine during the war now shrunk in response to the preferences of reciprocating nation-states and Britain's evolving political relationships with territories and countries within and outside of the Commonwealth. These challenges varied in scale. On one end of the spectrum was the retraction of reciprocity with Belgium in 1922. This came as no surprise because Belgium had originally agreed to reciprocate only for the duration of the hostilities. The demands of Italy and the newly created Irish Free State did not so much undermine the influence of British medicine as underscore the political nature of reciprocity. Separately, they conditioned the continuation of reciprocal relations with Britain on replacing the British Order in Council—which facilitated the implementation of the reciprocity provisions of the 1886 Medical Amendment Act—with a bilateral agreement. This demand was more about the form of reciprocity than its substance. Neither agreement fundamentally altered the GMC's statutory authority in regulating admission to the medical register as originally set out in the Order in Council. For these two nation-states—one that had just come into existence after a prolonged civil war and the other now led by fascist nationalists—a bilateral agreement symbolized equality within the community of nations as much as the equality of professionals. For its part, Britain benefited as much as the other parties to the agreements. The creation of the Irish

Free State may have territorially shrunk the United Kingdom. But the continuation of the regulation of the Irish profession through the GMC preserved the boundaries of British medicine. It also ensured the continuation of economic and social ties in the archipelago. The agreement with Italy ensured that resident British nationals would have access to British doctors. Correspondingly, Italian doctors operating within the boundaries of British medicine in the world would not be subject to differential treatment.

On the opposite end of the spectrum, conflicts in the Commonwealth increasingly called into question the legal rationale for the enforcement of the rights of registered doctors with third country qualifications to practice in another reciprocating territory or country. For most of the 1920s, the GMC defended the rights of registered doctors to local registration. In fact, it prevailed upon the Privy Council to revoke reciprocity in several provinces in Canada that refused to repeal selective registration policies. In the case of New Zealand, however, the GMC reversed course. In 1927 a Privy Council legal opinion, originally solicited by the GMC, upheld the dominion's right to limit automatic registration to only those doctors on the register who qualified or received their primary qualification in the United Kingdom. The reversal reflected not only the constitutionally subordinate position of the GMC, but also Britain's changing relationship with white-dominated dominions. By the time of the legal opinion, Britain had conceded effective autonomy in international affairs to the dominions. The presumed entitlement of registered doctors from British territories or foreign countries infringed on the rights of new nation-states to regulate the management of their domestic markets. While the New Zealand opinion underscored the growing parity between the GMC and its dominion counterparts, this was not the case for India. On the contrary, there the council expanded its authority. Beginning in 1919, the council began regular inspections of university licensing bodies in India based on its discretionary authority to grant or withdraw full recognition of medical qualifications. Its intervention highlighted the ways in which the GMC's authority reflected political changes within British colonialism.

Reciprocating Countries on the Foreign List

Belgium

In early 1919 the prospects for continuing reciprocity with Belgium after the war were already in doubt. J. S. Boruchowitz, a registered British doctor, complained to GMC registrar Norman King about the difficulty in obtaining access to the medical market in spite of the existence of reciprocity between the countries.[1] At the direction of the executive committee, King met with the Belgian ambassador at the embassy in London and reminded him of the terms of reciprocity; he in turn pledged to refer the matter to the minister of arts and science. In Belgium, as in Britain, the state delegated to a competent authority the evaluation of the qualifications of all applicants seeking to legally practice medicine. Boruchowitz's application received a favorable recommendation from Belgium's Jury Central of Medicine. Still, neither Boruchowitz nor the executive committee was confident in the outcome of the process as the end of the war drew near. Their skepticism reflected not only their awareness of the resistance of the Belgian medical profession to the admission of foreign medical graduates but also the conditional nature of the 1915 royal decree.[2] For its part, the executive committee of the GMC adopted a resolution urging the Belgian minister to act in good faith under the terms of the wartime royal decree and hoped that "no difficulty will be placed in the way of Medical Practitioners registered in this country who desire to practice their profession in Belgium."[3]

Adding to the uncertainty surrounding the outcome of Boruchowitz's application was the probable defeat of new legislation in Belgium that would place reciprocity on an enduring postwar basis. This bill, introduced in the Belgian Parliament by the minister of arts and science, was closely followed in London. In his remarks before the GMC, council president MacAlister said that he hoped that "the experience of our hospitality to Belgian practitioners may lead to the admission of British practitioners to the privilege of practicing in Belgium on equitable terms."[4] But King's summary of his meeting with representatives at the Belgian Embassy hardly inspired much hope. Although embassy officials had recognized admission to the register in the United Kingdom for nationals during wartime, all licensed medical practitioners were now required to complete the six-year medical degree in Belgium. Nor was King optimistic about appealing directly to the Jury Centrale for an exemption for British doctors.[5] Ultimately, in the absence of legislation, relations between Britain and Belgium reverted to the prewar status. A footnote in a listing of registrable colonial and foreign medical degrees simply noted after the defeat of the bill that "Belgium no longer appears in this list as the Government of that country requires British practitioners to obtain a Belgian qualification."[6]

Kingdom of Italy

Until 1923 the right to unrestricted practice remained unchanged in Italy. Italian officials neither raised concerns about the existing terms of reciprocity nor threatened to terminate them. But relations with the former ally cooled in the wake of the peace settlement, which left Italy feeling deprived of territorial claims that reflected its aspiration to be a world power. This nationalist sentiment animated Italy's postwar foreign policy, including its relations with Britain.[7] After the Fascist Party, led by Benito Mussolini, came to power in 1922, the Italian government issued a new decree early in 1923 governing the practice of medicine domestically. This decree conditioned the right to practice on the possession of a medical diploma awarded by an Italian institution or the possession of a diploma from a country that reciprocated with Italy based on a special agreement.

The 1923 decree, which signaled a shift in Italy's management of its domestic medical market, made no immediate impression on the council. The Italian Ministry of Health's June notification did not include the decree itself. Believing that the Order in Council was sufficient or equivalent to a special agreement, the registrar acknowledged receipt. But the experience of a registered British doctor soon belied this assumption. In November of 1923, H. J. Spon, a licentiate of the Royal College of Physicians, requested permission to practice at Ospedaletti from the local medical board of Proto Maurizio, San Remo. Board president P. Filippi denied his request, noting that he must first obtain an Italian Medical Diploma.[8] Initially, Spon attributed this response to a misunderstanding. Provincial authorities were often unaware of the 1910 Order in Council regulating relations between registered doctors in Britain and Italy. But as Spon was to learn, the denial was more than simply an omission. The minister of the interior informed the British ambassador and Spon that the reciprocity as provided for in the 1910 Order in Council, which had been confirmed by Italian law, was no longer enforceable. In a letter to GMC registrar Norman King, Spon stated that he hoped that "steps will at once be taken to draw up an agreement in the interests of all British Medical Practitioners desiring to practice in Italy."[9]

Like Boruchowitz's experience in Belgium, Spon's plight underscored the politically contingent nature of reciprocity. In theory, its viability was subject to each country honoring the terms of equitable treatment. The right to practice was not automatic but was subject to the assessment of the qualifications by competent authorities in the host country as well as the conditions mandated by legislation. Implied in the 1910 Order in Council was the expectation that each reciprocating country would consult with the relevant authorities in Britain in the event of any statutory or legislative modifications that could affect the rights of existing or future practitioners legally entitled to practice medicine. While it is true that the Italian Ministry of Health had notified the council of the new decree, this notification took place only after the decree took effect. Any consultation would also be complicated by the division of responsibility between the Privy Council and the GMC. The former made the decision on behalf of the government to extend part 2 of the Medical Act of 1886 and the latter approved qualified foreign and colonial practitioners for registration for admission to the register. This division of responsibility gave the council no independent standing either to initiate consultation or to otherwise engage with foreign countries. The GMC therefore could only react to alleged infringements on the rights of registered doctors.[10]

At first glance, Spon's treatment appeared to warrant the retraction of reciprocity with Italy.[11] Yet the council did not pursue this course of action. Retaliatory action would have adversely affected established and future practitioners and perhaps angered British nationals traveling or residing in Italy. Also, Italy remained open to negotiating a "special relationship" treaty that included the basic terms of the Order in Council. This agreement would change the form but not the content of reciprocity. Negotiations conducted by the Foreign Office rapidly yielded a draft agreement. MacAlister was generally satisfied with the terms.

But even though this agreement would normalize relations in medicine with Italy, MacAlister was conscious that the reach of British medicine was politically elastic. The expansion and contraction of reciprocal relations in the empire had a direct impact on all doctors on the register, including those on the foreign and colonial lists. Even though the wartime emergency had spurred several provinces in Canada to reciprocate with Britain to defend the mother country, MacAlister did not assume that reciprocity would endure. For this reason, he stressed that the language of the agreements with these provinces should not exaggerate either the power of Britain to legislate on behalf of the dominions or the permanency of reciprocating relations. To accommodate changes in the relation of Britain with these and other countries, King proposed more general, rather than specific, language in the agreement: "Better, therefore say, from the outset, 'possessions or dominions, between which and Great Britain medical reciprocity exists.'"[12]

Irish Free State

The creation of the Irish Free State in 1922 explicitly called into question British medicine as a political construction. The outbreak of World War I in the spring of 1914 interrupted the ongoing political settlement of the Irish Question brokered by the British Liberal government and political representatives from Catholic and Protestant communities. But while the blueprint for Home Rule mollified union loyalists, it antagonized moderate nationalists and provoked Irish republicans. For a period of six years, Ireland was to be divided between a majority Catholic population in the south and a Protestant population in the ten counties of the north. With Britain distracted by events in Europe, republicans, who sought a unified independent nation-state, seized control of government buildings in Dublin in Easter 1916. Their proclamation of a provisional government proved to be short-lived. Suppressed within a week, some eighty rebels were tried and received death sentences, and fifteen were executed. Rather than diminishing public support for the nationalist cause—which originally only appealed to a minority of the Irish population—the swift justice increased it. During the 1918 election, the Irish republican Sinn Fein group gained the overwhelming majority of seats in Ireland. Refusing to take their seats in Westminster, Sinn Fein activists instead declared all of Ireland a republic and established its own governing assembly in Dublin. Anxious to preserve the integrity of the United Kingdom, Britain conceded independence to southern Ireland in 1921 while retaining Northern Ireland as part of the union. However, this plan hinged on southern Ireland swearing allegiance to the British Crown, which was refused. After a bitter civil war, a compromise was reached. Southern Ireland was granted dominion status and remained nominally within the Commonwealth. It was renamed the Irish Free State.

The creation of the Irish Free State created uncertainty about the future relationship of Irish medicine to the GMC. Would the existence of a new state necessarily cut the professional ties between Irish institutions and doctors and the GMC? Would Ireland establish an autonomous medical council of its own for the control of its national profession? Would university and nonuniversity licensing bodies continue to participate on the council and award registrable qualifications? The answers to these questions had political consequences. The withdrawal of the Irish Free State would shrink the widening boundaries of British medicine in the world. Doctors registered in Ireland would no longer enjoy registration rights in the dominions and possessions of the empire as well as in Italy and Japan. Conversely, doctors on the foreign and colonial lists would be prohibited from legally practicing medicine in the Irish Free State.

The Irish transition to legislative autonomy added to the uncertainty rather than diminishing it. The Southern Ireland Act provided for a transitional period for the provisional Irish government. During this period, the Irish government adopted orders that progressively limited the application of legislation passed by the British Parliament before the formation of the Free State. Until 1925 the status of the Medical Act was unclear. Although the Irish government requested continuation of the Medical Act during the interim period, it reminded the British Ministry of Health in January 1922 that their future effect was contingent upon whether "the Parliament of the Irish Free State or Northern Ireland saw fit to legislate for practitioners within their respective areas."[13] The promulgation of a general order in March 1924 became a source of concern because the schedule of continuing legislation did not include the Medical Act. The implication of this omission was clear enough: the GMC would cease to control the profession in Ireland.

The general order anticipated the decision of the Executive Council of the Irish Free State in August 1925 to sever ties with the GMC. As John

Fleetwood and others have noted, control over the national profession was informed by the politics of national autonomy. The 1927 Practitioners Act clarified Ireland's relation to the world of medicine. This act provided for an independent medical register for Ireland and empowered a national council to regulate medical education and discipline among doctors on its register.[14] Although the establishment of the council changed the relationship between Ireland and Britain, it did not sever the ongoing professional union. In contrast to other countries, Irish licensing bodies continued to be represented on the General Medical Council. To ensure the continuation of the movement of doctors between countries, representatives from the Irish Free State, Northern Ireland, and Britain negotiated a reciprocity agreement that was incorporated in the British 1927 Medical Act.[15] These arrangements simultaneously recognized political change in the constitutional configuration of the archipelago without disrupting the jurisdiction of British medicine. Doctors on the register in Ireland and those on the British register could practice throughout the United Kingdom.[16]

Throughout the protracted recasting of the British polity, the GMC was circumspect. It is not unreasonable to speculate that its preference was for the continuation of the status quo. British medicine had been constructed based on combining national professions within the archipelago under a single governing body. While the GMC had been in existence for more than fifty years, the withdrawal of Ireland could have precipitated its disintegration. This possibility did not become a reality. There was little evidence of widespread support within the Irish medical profession for an independent medical council. On the contrary, Irish university and nonuniversity institutions were represented on the council and their qualifications entitled Irish medical graduates to practice medicine throughout the archipelago and the empire, not to mention Italy and Japan. For his part, GMC president MacAlister was confident that Irish representatives on the council would "be trusted to let 'sleeping dogs' lie, lest worse befall."[17]

This agreement—along with the treaty with Italy—testified to the flexibility of British medicine. In preserving its territorial scope, the GMC oversight of doctors from participating countries was unchanged. These binding agreements introduced a political complication in the council's management of the register. Any action such as extending or withdrawing recognition or reciprocity from a dominion or territory would have direct implications for Italy and Ireland in terms of where their nationals could and could not practice and, correspondingly, impose an obligation on these participating countries to open (or close) their national markets to doctors on the register with third country qualifications.[18] The latter concern was rarely raised in either Italy or Ireland. But colonial authorities did voice this qualm on numerous occasions during the interwar period. As I discuss in the next section, Canada and New Zealand unilaterally challenged the assumption that the qualifications of a doctor on the foreign or colonial lists was equivalent to a doctor who qualified in the United Kingdom.

Reciprocating Territories in the British Commonwealth and Empire

Canada: Saskatchewan and Ontario, 1924–25

Between 1886 and 1919, the GMC interpreted the Medical Act to mean that all doctors on the register—whether they qualified in the United Kingdom or not—must be considered equally qualified. This interpretation originated in 1900 during deliberations over Italy's application for reciprocity with Britain. Anxious to retaliate against Italy for what it interpreted as differential treatment of British doctors, the council sought a legal basis for differential treatment of Italian doctors in the United Kingdom. However, once the Privy Council decided to extend the Medical Act to Italy, the council changed course. Indeed, it now provided a legal rationale for ensuring the unrestricted right of the practice of medicine in all reciprocating countries or territories of the Crown. In 1911 the council used this rationale to discourage Quebec from adopting legislation that closed off local registration to doctors on the register who did not qualify in the United Kingdom. Quebec revised its legislation. This did not necessarily mean that the underlying issue in Quebec or other provinces in the dominion had been solved—namely, the right to regulate access to their markets. To be sure, during the war the provinces subordinated local interests to the defense of the mother country. Saskatchewan and Ontario lost little time in asserting their prerogative to regulate access to their local medical markets when peacetime returned, however.

A. MacG. Young, the registrar of the College of Physicians of Saskatchewan, was candid in explaining the underlying motive of the province to selectively admit doctors from the register. "This was our original intention, but apparently the Act was improperly worded. It was never our intention to admit practitioners from any Province in Canada by obtaining a British Registration Certificate."[19] In response, GMC registrar King raised the prospect of ending reciprocity. Career opportunities in the United Kingdom and empire would be closed off to the province's graduates. The implied threat did little to intimidate Young. The benefits of reciprocity were uneven. "If that be your decision, we will be obliged to accept it, but I would respectfully suggest that the present arrangement is more in the interest of your registrants than ours, as practically none of our men register in Great Britain for the purpose of practicing there, and I am credibly informed that in the near future other Provinces will soon pass the same limitations as we have done, which will mean that reciprocity for the purpose of inter-provincial registration will be of no use to our registrants."[20]

With the argument of self-interest blunted, King next appealed to the wider political ramifications of the province's actions, namely undermining relations between Canada and the wider British Empire. The course intended by Saskatchewan, which privileged local interests, created a double standard. "Your proposed action amounts to procuring for Saskatchewan graduates the rights to practice throughout the Empire, while you deny the right to practice in Saskatchewan to registered graduates from other parts of the Empire." The consequences were not isolated to the province alone. "Secondly, if Saskatchewan as a Province ceases to recognize British registrations, and puts itself in the position of British Columbia, the other Provinces will be constrained in self-defense to adopt a similar course and the possibility of Dominion, and therefore inter-provincial communication, is effectively blocked."[21]

Ontario, like Saskatchewan, chafed under the terms of reciprocity. As early as 1922, it raised the possibility of restricting registration to registered doctors who qualified in the United Kingdom exclusively. Wilberforce Akins, registrar of the College of Physicians and Surgeons of Ontario, was reluctant to assume responsibility for doctors in the province who obtained registration by virtue of their inclusion on the Colonial List. In denying this request, the council sought to quiet the concerns of the college by describing its own due diligence. "One of the requirements laid down in the Act is that before registration here, the applicant must satisfy the Registrar of his good character, and the fear that undesirable persons may obtain registration here and thereby a right to claim registration in Ontario does not seem to be well-founded."[22] Rather than quieting concerns, the response reinforced the sense of power differentials.

In the opinion of the college, two cases involving doctors with dubious reputations highlighted the inability of the council to regulate the boundaries of British medicine. The GMC had erased Ernest Willis from the register for a felony conviction in Britain. Willis thereafter became a resident of Toronto and requested reinstatement on the British Register, which was granted. The second case involved Alfred Thomas Conville, a resident of Ontario who engaged in chiropractic or alternative medicine. The college registered Conville on the strength of the fact that his name was entered on the colonial list even though he had been operating and issuing certificates on behalf of his Mano-Therapy College. The presence of an alternative practitioner on the register called into question the GMC's oversight responsibility of regular medicine. The college also took exception to the fact that it was not notified of the irregular nature of either of these cases nor consulted about the special agreement with Italy, although that reciprocity would allow Italian certified doctors to now practice in Ontario.[23]

King's response stressed that the council's oversight was appropriate, mitigating the implication of unilateral action. He noted that consultation with the dominions was reserved for entering into reciprocity with new states and territories or "for matters of state; but the Privy Council and the Medical Council do not act without due consideration of all the circumstances which sometimes it might not be politic to circulate widely."[24] In the absence of any changes to Britain's obligations, there was no need to consult with territories with which it reciprocated. In regard to the registration of Wells and Conville, King pointed out that the council's decisions were shaped by the judgment of the local profession. As early as 1922 Willis had earned reinstatement. His residence in Ontario "had no bearing upon the restoration." He rehabilitated himself; restored his "good character," and received "testimonials from members of your College." Nor was the decision to register Conville problematic. Local practitioners Dr. John Ranson Howitt of the Medical School, London, Ontario, and Dr. Adam Scott Beuglas, a physician in Hamilton, vouched for him. Finally, King reminded Aikins that the British medical market would be closed off to Ontario graduates in the event of the rescinding of reciprocity: "Since the establishment of reciprocity 777 practitioners have registered in virtue of Ontario qualifications. Of these 162 were registered during the War and the remainder from the beginning of 1919. The Council has no means of ascertaining how many practitioners have registered in Ontario in virtue of registration here, but it would be surprising if the number were at all equivalent. If this assumption is correct . . . it appears that the Ontario practitioners will be the greatest sufferers in the long run."[25] Reciprocity was rescinded in these two provinces and others. In less than five years, Britain halved the number of provinces it reciprocated with in Canada.

New Zealand, 1924–27

Shortly after the Privy Council rescinded reciprocity with Saskatchewan, New Zealand notified the council of its own amended 1924 Medical Act. This act granted the New Zealand Medical Council the authority to register only those practitioners who qualified in the United Kingdom.[26] This discretionary authority excluded practitioners on the foreign list from automatic registration. More so than the actions of the Canadian provinces, this legislation was a major source of concern. New Zealand was the first dominion to begin reciprocating with the United Kingdom, and its relations with the GMC had been largely without perturbations. The example of a reliable dominion like New Zealand challenging aspects of the British Medical Act raised the prospect of other dominions unilaterally redefining the boundaries of British medicine in ways that complicated the GMC's relations with foreign countries. King reluctantly put the New Zealand Medical Council on notice about the consequences of a law deemed not just. The council would have no other choice but to recommend to the Privy Council the revocation of reciprocity.[27] New Zealand medical graduates would not be able to register as a matter of right, but be forced to requalify in the United Kingdom. King closed his letter on a conciliatory tone, hoping that the amended act not be implemented. "The Council does not propose to suspend the registration of New Zealand practitioners while the subject is under discussion," he wrote.[28]

Coming on the heels of a series of revocation recommendations and growing official concern about the implications of Britain's agreements with Italy and the Irish Free State, even MacAlister felt the need to solicit legal advice. In requesting an opinion of the law officers of the Privy Council, MacAlister requested answers to two questions: (1) What is the true construction and import of part 2 of the Medical Act, 1886; and (2) what is the precise meaning of the expression of registered medical practitioner of the United Kingdom?[29] Given the certainty with which the council had enforced the binding nature of the terms of reciprocity in the recent past, the law opinion came as a surprise.[30] At issue was the meaning of the phrase "registered medical practitioner of the United Kingdom" in relation to doctors on the foreign and colonial lists. Were they one and the same or different? Part 2 of the Medical Act provided for admission to the register in the United Kingdom for doctors either from reciprocating British territories or foreign countries. There was, however, no specific provision for doctors on the colonial and foreign lists to practice medicine of the United Kingdom. The reference to doctors referred only to "registered medical practitioners in the United Kingdom." Up to this point, the council had defended the rights of doctors with third country qualifications based on the assumption that all doctors on the register were subject to the same rights and responsibilities. Rejecting this implied authority, the law officer reached a wholly different determination. "In our opinion the phrase 'registered medical practitioners of the United Kingdom' is used to denote persons on the register who are neither 'colonial practitioners' nor 'foreign practitioners.'" Only registered British doctors had standing or at least had the benefit of the good offices or protection of the British government while doctors on the foreign and colonial lists of the register were subject to the vagaries of "local law." "The extent to which any local law in the case of British possessions or foreign law limits or forbids the right of registered medical practitioners of the United Kingdom to practice in the British possession or foreign country concerned is a matter for consideration by His Majesty in deciding whether the privileges of practicing afforded by such British possession or foreign country are or are not just."[31]

This opinion raised "political and executive difficulty." Up to this point the binding nature of reciprocity provided colonial territories and foreign countries either with an incentive to participate or a disincentive to withdraw. If anything, the decision of provincial authorities in Canada that sought to restrict registration to doctors on the United Kingdom register seemed to be the legally appropriate move. By contrast, the actions of the GMC appeared to reflect a gross misunderstanding of the medical act or political brinksmanship. Neither interpretation reflected well on either the GMC or the Privy Council. At the same time, this new perspective of a narrow application of the act raised further complications in regard to the recent bilateral agreement with Italy.[32] The government now refused to enforce the reciprocity provisions on Italy's behalf in the dominion. "The Dominions Office have also been advised that so long as recognition in New Zealand is not accorded to Italian practitioners on the Foreign List of the United Kingdom register, the understanding given by the United Kingdom in the agreement with Italy cannot, if the case arises, be carried out." The implications for third countries became immediately clear. An inquiry from the Italian counsel general spurred consultations between the Foreign Office and the Privy Council to coordinate their efforts.

> It may be quite true, as the General Medical Council say, that reciprocity in fact exists with the Union of South Africa, for instance but it is quite clear from the legal position disclosed as a result of the controversy with New Zealand that we are not in a position to enforce reciprocity as regards foreign practitioners on the Medical Register should a Dominion or any parts of it object in any particular case and we might possibly weaken our position with Italy if we had informed them that the necessary reciprocity existed under the agreement as regards such places. If, however, we can avoid it, we are very anxious not to stir up a hornet's nest by opening the question with all places concerned.[33]

Both the council and the Privy Council shared an interest in minimizing the political fallout of this opinion.[34] The legal opinion reinforced the growing autonomy of the dominions that had accelerated after the war. In 1926 the Imperial Conference, which comprised Britain and self-governing dominions, explicitly acknowledged dominions as "autonomous Communities within the British empire, equal in status . . . unified by means of a common allegiance to the Crown, and freely associated as members of the British Commonwealth." An extension of their autonomy included the right of dominions to conduct their own foreign policy and enter into international agreements. The government was loath to challenge this trend. The imminent Imperial Conference scheduled for the autumn of 1930 provided a serviceable opportunity to assign responsibility for the shift in the rights of doctors on the foreign and colonial lists while the council notified New Zealand via the Privy Council that it remained in good standing.[35]

The privileged place of national medicine within the British imperial nation-state had now come full circle. Harnessing Britain's imperial authority, the GMC had long used its control over the medical register to privilege British national medicine and its medical graduates by negotiating reciprocal agreements with foreign countries without consulting its territories or dominions. As of 1930, the dominions were entitled to impose differential standards and to prohibit the registration of medical graduates who qualified outside of Britain. Politically, this opinion reinforced for national medicine what the 1931 Statute of Westminster—the parliamentary sanction of the 1926 Imperial Conference—did for the successor states of the empire: parity.

In British India, parity proved to be far more nominal than real. Just as Britain sought to manage the political process of Indian self-government in the wake of World War I, the GMC began asserting oversight over medical education in the subcontinent. Over the following decade, the council justified its withdrawal of recognition of Indian medical degrees as a spur for the establishment of uniform standards of medical education. This justification exhibited the imperial logic of British medicine, in which British medicine is treated as a universal expression of modern medicine, in contrast to the heterogeneity of medical education in India. Following this logic, colonial autonomy in medicine could only be achieved through conforming to the norms of British medicine.

Medical Dyarchy: The GMC and British India

Britain's changing political relationship with India as its preeminent colonial possession spurred the council to redefine its oversight over medical education in the colony. Prior to World War I, Britain faced a growing tide of nationalist aspiration and protest. The establishment of the Indian National Congress in 1885 and the rise of militant Hinduism provided sites for Indians to channel their criticism against British colonialism. The 1908 boycott of British-made goods challenged Britain's moral authority and exhibited the potential impact of mass action. While these and other developments attracted the attention of the government of India, they did not pose an immediate or existential threat to British rule. The urban orientation of political mobilization plus the uneasy coexistence of Hindu and Muslim communities enabled officials to manage events through a policy of concession and repression while exacerbating communal differences. Britain's unilateral declaration of war on behalf of the empire and Indian congressional support for the defense of the mother country certainly interrupted nationalist activity but did not end the Indian demand for self-government. When peacetime returned, the Satyagraha protest movement, led by Mohandas Gandhi, mobilized a vast number of nonelites in rural and urban communities alike. Combining nonviolent protest, civil disobedience, and a rejection of western values, this movement strengthened the scope and scale of anticolonial nationalism.

Even though Britain emerged as a victor from World War I, it was militarily and financially overextended. Seeking to prolong rule, the secretary of state for India, Edwin Montagu, in 1917 outlined Britain's commitment to eventual self-government for India. An early installment of this policy involved the devolution of power from an all-India or central administration, controlled by British personnel, to provincial governments that would be directly elected. The areas that fell under provincial administration included medical education. This had implications for the composition of the faculty of university-affiliated medical schools. Before devolution, the all-Indian medical administration influenced the selection of principal and professor positions in medical schools. Candidates were nominated by the Government of India based on the advice of the director-general of the India Medical Service (IMS) or its provincial-level representatives such as surgeons general or inspectors general of civil hospitals. The policy of provincialization recast the terms of control over the gateways to western medicine. When writing to his counterpart in New Zealand to underscore the council's regulation of the register, GMC registrar Norman King pointed out how events in India necessitated greater vigilance. "With regard to India, the position has recently changed somewhat, and, instead of practically the whole of the teachers being Europeans and members of the Indian Medical Service, the staff of many Universities is now largely composed of Indians, of whom many have not studied out of India."[36]

King's concern about medical education in India was a departure for the GMC since the application of the Medical Act in 1892. Between 1892 and 1921, the council successively recognized the primary medical qualifications of several provincial universities: Bombay (1892); Calcutta, Madras, and Punjab (1893); Allahabad (1914); and Lucknow (1921). In light of the institutional and social ties between Britain and British India, recognition was not necessarily unusual. These universities were modeled on British institutions much like other universities in the empire. As a matter of fact, before the 1886 Medical Act the council had approved of the general education certificates and university degrees of Bombay and Calcutta for satisfying premedical studies. British-trained doctors for the most part staffed the faculty. Such appointments were among the most prized civil appointments for doctors in the IMS while racial bars in the service limited competition from western-trained Indian doctors.[37]

For the most part, the council's interaction with university degree- or diploma-granting bodies was limited to processing requests for the recognition of registrable degrees or diplomas. Section 13 of the 1886 Medical Act provided for recognition so long as the degree or diploma furnished "a sufficient guarantee of the possession of the requisite knowledge and skill for the efficient practice of medicine, surgery and midwifery."[38] Once recognized, the council had no oversight of these qualifications in reciprocating countries or territories. While part 1 of the Medical Act empowered the council to visit examinations and to inspect medical schools in the United Kingdom, no such provision was made for these activities beyond the archipelago. This omission recognized the authority of reciprocating governments and their delegated bodies to oversee medical education. It is likely for this reason that the council did not interact with university and nonuniversity licensing bodies or communicate with them about new regulations or policies governing medical education in the United Kingdom.

The recognition of qualifications affiliated with Indian universities created a steep threshold for institutional eligibility. The council was therefore loath to recognize qualifications from nonuniversity entities such as the membership and proposed fellowship diplomas from the College of Surgeons and Physicians of Bombay presidency. Created after the passage of the Bombay Registration Act in 1912, the college was the first nonuniversity medical body dedicated to regulating western medicine in India. Presided over by the surgeon general of the presidency, it regulated the medical profession through the maintenance of a voluntary medical register and by monitoring examinations administered by provincial medical schools and independent colleges. Admission to the college was open to doctors holding either a registrable degree as recognized by the GMC as well as those to those without such qualifications.

This open membership was designed to reconcile the perverse effects of the privileged place of British qualifications within colonial India. Although Bombay and other jurisdictions could boast of registrable university degrees, the production of western-trained doctors in India was well below the needs of the colonial government. Over the course of the century, a large number of nonuniversity-affiliated colleges arose that supplemented university-affiliated medical schools. There was a significant distinction between these graduates. Lacking a registrable qualification, graduates of the nonuniversity-affiliated institutions were only eligible for the native or subordinate medical service within the IMS. While this large pool of medical labor enabled the colonial government to deliver health care beyond the limited capacity of the European-dominated IMS, these doctors' marginal status both reinforced the racial stratification of western medicine and checked the growth of an independent profession. The college proposed offering diplomas to personnel in the subordinate service, giving them the opportunity to augment their training and credentialing while also promising to upgrade the standards of medical education in India. They asked the GMC to recognize their diplomas.

The council declined the college's request. Given the pool of medical personnel, the council feared that the diplomas would undermine the credibility of British medicine. There were inadequate safeguards to ensure quality control, such as the possession of preliminary education for all candidates for the membership examination and the completion of an articulated course of studies before sitting for more advanced examinations. Even after the college agreed to amend its regulations, the council still deemed the diplomas insufficient. When requesting reconsideration, the India Office stressed the training needs of India as a compelling rationale for recognition:

> The Government of India feel that it is very important that the diplomas should be registrable in the United kingdom, being of the opinion that they are equal in every respect to the medical degrees granted at Bombay University. Non-recognition not only affects the general value of the diplomas, but prejudices candidates from the College in regard to the Indian Medical Service. Incidentally it practically debars a military assistant surgeon from obtaining a qualification registerable in the United Kingdom and serious handicaps him in his relations with the civil assistant surgeons.[39]

Rather than becoming more accommodating to the local circumstances, the council became more unyielding. "The Executive Committee," according to a resolution, "are of opinion that the courses of study and examination prescribed for these qualifications do not furnish such a guarantee as the Medical Act, 1886, requires of the possession of the requisite knowledge and skill for the efficient practice of medicine, surgery, and midwifery *in this country*." The resolution underscored the position that British standards were not to be sacrificed for the benefits of the unique conditions in India: "The committee express no view as to the suitability for Indian conditions and requirements. They recognize that in some respects the Governing Body or the College has amended its regulations in the direction of greater stringency of examination; but it appears to the Committee that it is still possible for Licentiates trained as 'Military Assistant Surgeons,' who have, in addition to their incomplete course of study and examination for that grade, taken certain supplementary courses out of due order in the curriculum, to procure the qualifications of the College."[40] The resolution added that "the relation of 'candidates from the College' to the Indian Medical Service and to Civil Assistant Surgeons does not appear to the Committee to have any necessary connection with the question of registration by the General Medical Council, and the Committee do not see it to be their duty to have regard to such relation in determining the latter question."[41]

Underlying the rationale of the council's decision was an explicit articulation of the standard of medicine necessary for recognition of medical diplomas: Britain. Before the postwar period, the geographical and social meaning of the phrase "requisite knowledge and skill for the efficient practice of medicine, surgery, and midwifery" remained implied. But in practice, the government's extension of reciprocity and the council's subsequent recognition of medical qualifications for admission to the register was grounded in the presumptive equality of white male medical professionals and the parity of dominions within the territorial jurisdiction of the British Empire. India was equivalent so long as registered British doctors dominated the medical faculties and Western-trained Indian doctors inhabited the margins of British medicine in the colony. Although the council lacked the authority to inspect medical schools in reciprocating territories, these conditions provided the necessary assurance that Indian qualifications satisfied "the requisite knowledge and skill for the efficient practice of medicine surgery, and midwifery *in this country*."[42]

By 1919 the council's position had changed. MacAlister requested information about the courses and instruction in midwifery from all Indian universities.[43] The request from the council was unprecedented. It amounted to an expansion of its authority in relationship to licensing bodies in reciprocating countries or territories, the first since the passage of the 1886 Medical Act. Until this time, the council had generally managed the register in two ways: reviewing the medical qualifications for recognition from licensing bodies or defending the rights of doctors on the register who faced differential treatment. As discussed above, the leverage of the council was diminished when dealing with countries where British nationals and practitioners lived and worked, such as Italy, or in territories with independent professions, such as New Zealand. Preserving the rights of the former strengthened the negotiating hand of hosting countries, while well-defined medical markets in the latter case enabled territories to forgo employment opportunities in the empire that were associated with being registered. While the recourse available to the council with noncompliant territories was to revoke reciprocity, in the case of India the council went further and decided to threaten to withhold recognition. Dissatisfied with the replies from Indian universities, the council issued an ultimatum: either bring training into compliance or face the loss of recognition.

This was provocative in light of Montagu's announcement about self-government in India. It highlighted the imperial nature of the authority of British medicine. Without registerable degrees, the IMS would be closed off to Indian medical graduates while leaving them eligible only for the subordinate service, if not the vagaries of private practice. Rather than promoting Indianization, the council's action would doom Indian doctors to a second-class status. The stakes for medical schools were no less consequential. Their diplomas would be no better than those of nonuniversity medical colleges. On behalf of university officials, Montagu requested additional time.[44] The legislative assembly concurred but not before Madras member Bahadur C. S. Subramaniam suggested that the secretary of state discontinue recruiting in Britain for the IMS or make an Indian qualification a condition of admission to the service.[45] In seeking to privilege the institutions and qualifications of India, Subramaniam attempted a strategy that was available to white-settled dominions. But the IMS was one of the reserved portfolios in the policy of decentralization; that is, it remained controlled by the all-India administration and was predominately staffed by Europeans.

The secretary of state for India and MacAlister reached a compromise: a joint inspection. Under this compromise, Norman Walker, a member of the GMC, would conduct an inspection of all universities and report. Lieutenant colonel and deputy-general of the IMS Richard Needham, a government of India appointee, would accompany Walker. During a six-week period, Walker and Needham toured universities in Bombay, Punjab, Delhi, Lucknow, and Calcutta.[46] The results of the tour were contained in a report that consisted of a university-by-university assessment with recommendations for recognition. In his narrative, Walker framed the council's concern in terms of Indian particularity—that is, how local conditions checked the progress of conformity to British standards and thereby necessitated intervention. "Although legally speaking the relation of India to the General Medical Council is the same as that of any other reciprocating country or British Possession overseas, it is impossible to ignore the fact that practically the relation has exceptional features in regard to obstetric education."[47] Underlying Indian particularity was its opposite: British medicine as a universal representation of western medicine. Rather than regarding local conditions as constitutive of British medicine, this binary lens rendered them as characteristics of the incomplete development of India.

Walker's report therefore dismissed or attempted to explain away any reference to the uneven power relationship that simultaneously reproduced the authority of British medicine and Indian difference. He conceded that universities were held responsible for regulations concerning midwifery even though the council did not notify them of changes. At the same time, he rebuffed claims of the council applying differential standards. When reminded of statements in the British medical press—even by members of the council—on the reform of midwifery that favorably compared the methods at Bombay, Calcutta, and Madras to several schools in Britain, he minimized their import. "I replied that India was not concerned with the opinion of individual members of the Council expressed in debate, but must accept the considered judgment of the Council as a whole, and I turned the attack by commenting on the fact that they evidently had fuller and more detailed knowledge of what was going on than one would have expected when they complained of insufficient notice of the Council's Regulations."[48] He also characterized as irrational the association of the threat to withdraw recognition with the practice of limiting access to the IMS to Indian doctors. "The Indian practitioners have a deep-rooted suspicion that the requirement of a registrable qualification for admission to the Indian Medical Service is, in fact, a plot to preserve that Service for Europeans." Walker attempted to deflect this "suspicion" by pointing out that "the Council have nothing whatever to do with the conditions off admission to the Indian Medical Service, but was merely discharging its Statutory Duties under Part 2 of the 1886 Act."[49]

Walker's discussion of individual universities simultaneously reinforced the disinterestedness of the council and justified the need for its oversight. At Madras and Bombay, where IMS personnel or European doctors served as the principal of the college or occupied chairs of midwifery, Walker declared himself satisfied with the curriculum and the number of cases available to students, and only recommended improved coordination among the different faculty groups at Bombay. By contrast, at Calcutta, he was concerned by the large number of students relative to the limited supply of cases. This concern was amplified at the recently affiliated Carmichael Medical College, staffed mainly by Indian doctors. Walker did report, though, that he was impressed by the earnest attention of the university authorities and medical faculty to find a solution. At Punjab and Lucknow, cases were in short supply. By linking this deficiency in medical education to the practice of purdah (or the spatial separation of women from men to promote modesty in an observant Muslim's life), Walker reiterated a well-worn trope of the backwardness of Indian civilization. "[In Lahore] the Purdah nashin system dominates the situation, and labor cases are very rarely attended by men. The rest of the subjects in the medical curriculum, are exceedingly well organized and taught in Labor, but the Faculty of Medicine seem to have gradually yielded to the custom of the country and have taken less and less interest in the subject of Practical Midwifery." Lucknow laws were little different. "Its hospital, laboratories are all very well equipped, but the 'custom of the country' in respect of midwifery is the same as Lahore, and there is no early prospect of change." The willingness of both colleges to undertake corrective action not only validated Walker's criticism, but also the salutary impact of his visit. Walker successfully lobbied the minister of education to support Punjab students so that they would be able to complete their practical midwifery at Madras. Even before his arrival there, Lucknow had made similar arrangements.[50]

Even though Walker was broadly satisfied, his recommendations imposed a tight accountability regime on university licensing bodies in the future. He recommended conditional recognition on a year-by-year basis for all universities, except Madras. Even though he did not visit Madras University, he was confident in the guarantee of their qualifications. "The fact that the Indian Medical Service sends those of its officers who are deficient in these subjects to Madras for instruction in them is for the Council almost sufficient evidence that the possession of the degree of that University guarantees a knowledge of Medicine, Surgery, and Midwifery sufficient to ensure their efficient practice."[51] Continued recognition for all other qualifications was conditioned on the outcome of annual inspection. To this end, Walker proposed that the Government of India appoint Needham to conduct a follow-up tour. "I suggest that the Government of India should be advised to approach the General Medical Council with the proposal that the services of Colonel R. A. Needham, deputy general of the Indian Medical Service, who accompanied me throughout my tour and was present at, and is fully cognizant of all that took place at, the meetings in connection therewith, should be accepted as those of the Inspector hereafter proposed."[52]

The council endorsed Walker's recommendations, and the Government of India appointed Needham as the official inspector of universities for 1923. For his part, President MacAlister defended the proposed inspection regime in terms of the council's statutory duty to protect the British public. During an address to the council, he insisted that the council's responsibility was to ensure training that related to the domestic medical market in the United Kingdom, not accommodating local conditions or needs. This responsibility justified local inspection and the withdrawal of recognition from licensing bodies that either failed or refused to comply.[53]

The compliance of Indian universities to the inspection regime validated the rationale of the council. The inspection regime itself was modeled on the United Kingdom. The 1886 Medical Act empowered the council to inspect facilities and appoint visitors to observe examinations at university and nonuniversity licensing bodies in the United Kingdom. Needham was briefed on domestic inspection before his first tour of Indian universities in 1923.[54] Until 1924 all but one university provided Needham with information, entry to facilitates, and access to examinations. Calcutta University refused to admit Needham to its examinations. The syndicate reminded him and the council that degree recognition was not part of the extension of part 2 of the Medical Act and as such "can never mean inspection either of the colleges or of the examinations held under the auspices of the University."[55] Unwilling to be drawn into a debate about the council's right to inspect, Calcutta became the first university to be stripped of recognition.[56] The loss of recognition had material consequences for existing and prospective medical students. They were ineligible for IMS appointments. Calcutta's independence was short-lived. In 1927 it sought recognition from the council.

The interactions with Calcutta displayed the council's authority and political will. But the example of Calcutta, no less than the inspections themselves, proved inadequate to maintaining the council's desired standards of British medicine in India. Walker said as much in his second and final report in 1927.[57] At the request of the secretary of state for India, Walker reviewed medical schools and provided an overview of medical education. In the five years since the first inspection Walker noted progress, particularly in the curriculum and physical facilities. He was troubled, however, by the quality of medical education. The decline in the presence of Europeans or personnel from the IMS on faculties continued with the devolution of medical administration to provinces. In some colleges, Europeans and IMS personnel were prohibited from serving. In others "unofficial Indian gentlemen" held teaching positions alongside IMS personnel. In Lucknow and Patna, Europeans, even those with degrees from Oxford, Cambridge, and Aberdeen Universities were reduced to five-year contract appointments.[58]

Walker painted a bleak picture of the local divergence from a British standard of medical education. India lacked the depth of talent of Britain. While some colleges employed hospital attending doctors to supplement their teaching faculty—as was the practice in the United Kingdom—the results could not be more different. "I came across instances in India where men had been appointed professors whose teaching experience is small, whose training as teachers has been short and sometimes carried out under conditions not likely to give the best results,"[59] said Walker. Nor was the quality of medical students equivalent. The students were too young. Students could enter the university as young as fourteen and enter upon medical studies at sixteen. Nor was academic preparation the sole basis of admission. The demand for spots in medical schools far exceeded supply. A culture of financial incentives too often influenced admission decisions. Even for those who were admitted, the mismatch of the language of instruction (English) and the vernacular of the students meant that students were "unable to follow intelligently conversational English in which clinics are usually conducted." Walker volunteered that students compensated with memorizing texts. But, memorization was not a substitute for the ability to take a case history and examine a patient. "On this may be founded the common statement that though good in written examination work the Indian student is deficient in his knowledge of practical work,"[60] he said.

Like British rule itself, the effect of provincialization set in motion forces that the council could not control. Even with regular visits and reports from the government of India inspector and the threat of the withdrawal of recognition, local conditions exposed the limits of the council's authority, not to mention the inadequacy of western medicine that Britain had introduced to India. Before World War I, the council was indifferent to Indian medical education. But once Indians assumed positions of power, indifference quickly turned to new attempts at control. Within five years, even Walker conceded the futility of the council's efforts. At the same time, he did not deem India as wholly lost to British medicine. On the contrary, Walker proposed the creation of an all-India medical council.[61] Given the bleak portrait of Indian medical education, less control from London seemed unlikely to reverse the trends he described. For this reason, Walker's recommendation was a political solution rather than a practical one. In light of the New Zealand legal opinion, the proposed council preserved the fiction of British medicine as a voluntary association of dominions dedicated to common standards of medicine and led by Britain. This fiction was only possible, however, if qualified colonial medical graduates from India did not seek to practice medicine in the United Kingdom. Otherwise, the council would have to confront a major challenge posed by the globalization of British medicine: mediating the aspiration for homogeneity within national medicine and the reality of racial heterogeneity inside its territorial boundaries.

Acknowledging the challenge of arriving at a legislative solution that provided for an all-India medical council, Walker proposed transitional machinery that consisted of a commissioner of medical qualifications and standards. Reporting to the Department of Public Health, the commissioner would continue and expand upon the work of Needham. Under these conditions, "the General Medical Council would willingly accept such an Official as their Visitor, and his regular reports would be of much assistance in determining whether or not recognition could be continued or accorded."[62] This proposal faced hurdles for several years. The government preferred visits by senior members of the IMS and the provinces were reluctant to submit to an all India medical council. Bringing matters to a head was the decision by the Legislative Assembly to deny funding for another round of visits by Needham. In the absence of an annual report, the council warned India of the imminent withdrawal of recognition. As Roger Jeffrey has noted, withdrawal led provinces to reverse "their stand, recognizing that potential control from New Delhi was preferable to actual control from London."[63]

A bill for the creation of the medical council of India was introduced in June 1932 and became law in 1934. In several ways, the new Medical Council of India (MCI) resembled the GMC. Its membership consisted of nominated members (one for each provincial government and four for the central government) and elected members (one for each university and one for each provincial register). Similarly, the function of the council was to maintain uniform minimum standards of the higher qualifications while at the same time coordinating recognition of these qualifications among provinces. Like the Medical Council of Canada, the MCI did not replace the jurisdiction of provincial medical bodies. As a result, Indian graduates of provincial institutions were not entitled to unrestricted practice outside of the province from which they received their primary qualification. Yet the MCI coordinated the recognition of medical qualifications with countries or territories within the empire that reciprocated with India.

The implementation of the act reinforced the unbalanced position of India in relation to the GMC and other reciprocating dominions. The council was embedded in the structure of the colonial state. It consisted of thirty-eight members. Seven (18 percent) represented university licensing bodies, fifteen (39 percent) government nominees (central and provincial) and representatives of general practitioners eight (21 percent). This composition contrasted with the GMC itself, in which university and nonuniversity licensing bodies accounted for twenty-seven (71 percent), government nominees five (13 percent), and six (16 percent) representatives of registered practitioners.[64] The influence of the state extended to the appointment of the council president. Under the implementation regulations, the governor general appointed the director-general of the IMS as the inaugural president. This appointment, which was endorsed by the council, symbolized the historical role of the IMS in providing oversight for medical education. Similarly, the appointment of John MacCrae, a former GMC Inspector of Medical Examination, as secretary to the MCI underscored the enduring influence of the GMC. MacCrae held the position of secretary along with that of medical inspector, thereby combining the post of inspector with a salaried position.[65]

Conclusion

On the eve of the World War II, the boundaries of British medicine remained as extensive as ever. They comprised the United Kingdom and the new Free State of Ireland, the dominions and the dependent territories of the Commonwealth, and foreign countries Italy and Japan. The outward continuity masked a two-decade period of tension and change in British medicine.

The interwar period exposed the politically contingent nature of the influence of British medicine as local interests increasingly collided with imperial interests. This was particularly the case concerning the rights of doctors on the foreign and colonial list of the medical register to practice in countries and dominions reciprocating with the United Kingdom. The council had interpreted the relevant sections of the Medical Act broadly. Where the act specified that all registered British doctors were entitled to practice in reciprocating countries and dominions, the council construed registered doctors to include those on the foreign and colonial list. A combination of constitutional changes within the United Kingdom and challenges within the Commonwealth exposed the contradictions between the language of the act and the interpretation of the council. The formation of the Irish Free State in 1920 complicated the relationship of the council with the new country. The council's jurisdiction was now subject to the political preferences of the new state. While an agreement with the Free Sate and Northern Ireland perpetuated the jurisdiction of the council, it created uncertainty about the rights of reciprocating countries with Britain to practice medicine in Ireland. Did the agreement between two states necessarily extend to other reciprocating countries?

Meanwhile legislative action in the provinces of the federated dominion of Canada and New Zealand challenged the British register as a gateway to their medical markets. Even though several provinces agreed to reciprocate with the United Kingdom during the war, this did not mean that they embraced open borders within the dominion or with the worldwide community within the orbit of British medicine. Ontario and Quebec, among others, regarded third party reciprocity as a route that diluted control over their medical markets. Legislation restricting local registration to those on the British register who qualified in the United Kingdom was designed to address this concern. Appeals from the GMC register and council president to the commonwealth spirit and economic benefits associated with reciprocity proved to be in vain. Similar legislation in New Zealand in 1924 led the council to call for a legal opinion from the law officers of the Privy Council. Their 1927 decision upheld the right of reciprocating countries to limit registration to those who qualified in the United Kingdom. This decision recast the nature of the relationship between the GMC and counterparts. It was based on parity. India, however, was a different matter. While the Medical Council of India provided India-wide oversight of medical education, the influence of the Government of India and the GMC was significant and circumscribed a nationally independent institution.

The conflicts that characterized the interwar period captured the underlying tensions at the heart of reconciling national medicine in an imperial context. In theory, opening the register provided a mechanism for managing British medicine among colonial territories. In practice, colonial professions sought to control access to their markets to privilege their institutions and graduates or otherwise preserve the homogeneity of their professions. The New Zealand legal opinion certainly reflected Britain's recognition of the autonomy of dominions to govern their internal and external affairs. At the same time, the principle of equity for foreign and colonial doctors was for all intents and purposes ended. In exchange for ensuring that British practitioners would retain their rights to practice medicine legally in reciprocating countries and dominions, the GMC accepted the differential treatment of doctors based on country of primary qualification.

Chapter Four

The International Crisis of World War II and the Differential Treatment of Overseas-Trained Doctors, 1933–48

Introduction

As the interwar landscape of international politics rapidly shifted from the threat to the reality of a second global war, the influence of British medicine was once again challenged, from the plight of Jewish medical refugees in the United Kingdom before the war to the wartime need to supplement the domestic supply of doctors. The register proved to be a rather flexible instrument in accommodating overseas-trained and refugee doctors, in large part due to the multiple points of entry to the medical market, yet the conditions under which refugee doctors were admitted to the register and legally entitled to practice medicine were not identical. Institutional interests and national needs shaped whether or not the register differentiated overseas doctors from domestic doctors in ways that assimilated or marginalized them in the community of British medicine. As I will show in this chapter, the experience the council gained in internationalizing the register during wartime established a precedent for a new postwar registration category for overseas doctors. Temporary registration, which became available with the passage of the 1948 Medical Act, combined access to medical labor with restrictions on where and how long overseas doctors could practice medicine in the United Kingdom.

More so than any other group, Jewish medical refugees from the early 1930s on were vulnerable to differential treatment. Fleeing brutal persecution in Germany, Austria, and later Italy, Britain only permitted a fraction to enter as aliens. Stateless and subject to Home Office employment restrictions, these doctors and medical students who sought to practice medicine in the United Kingdom had few choices beyond requalification. As Kenneth Collins and other scholars have documented, nonuniversity licensing bodies in England and Ireland were resistant to calls from the government to accommodate more Jewish aliens.[1] At a moment when the economy was struggling to recover from depression, any increase in the number of doctors beyond replacement levels raised competition anxieties. When the refugee crisis appeared to grow rather than decline, accommodation was seen as a precedent that was liable to change the ethnic composition of British medicine. While the licensing bodies relented and agreed to a fixed quota of refugees from Germany and Austria, they also prolonged the qualifying period of residence in Britain from three to five years (with the exception of the Scottish licensing bodies, who kept the qualifying period the same). The discriminatory treatment of refugees continued after they qualified and were admitted to the register. Their rights to practice—that is, location, clinical setting, and duration—were curtailed because of their immigration status as aliens. Meanwhile, the BMA was vigilant in insisting on Home Office enforcement of these restrictions.

Just as the register could be an instrument of exclusion, it also functioned as an instrument of inclusion. The outbreak of World War II in 1939 heralded an immediate expansion of the territorial reach of the register. Drawing a lesson from World War I, policy makers understood well that Britain lacked the domestic supply of doctors to meet the massive personnel requirements needed to support an ever-expanding war at home and beyond. Rather than relying on negotiating bilateral reciprocity agreements with each country, the War Cabinet promulgated a series of temporary registration orders that extended full recognition to foreign doctors to practice medicine for the duration of the war. These orders served an equally important political purpose: wartime propaganda. They removed a barrier so as to make it easier for doctors from neutral countries such as the United States and Canada and belligerent countries like Germany, Italy, and Japan to support the British war effort either in a military or civilian capacity. Their participation displayed the scope of international support for Britain's war effort. However, although wartime necessity opened the register, this did not mean that all foreign doctors were treated equally. Britain did harness the labor of alien doctors from belligerent countries but with highly restrictive conditions. They were permitted to practice medicine in designated hospitals or other clinical settings while under the watchful eyes of British medical and nursing personnel. Their fitness to practice was therefore subject to the vagaries of the wartime political climate as much as it was to their professional qualifications.

Selective Admission to the Register: The GMC and Foreign Jewish Medical Refugees, 1933–35

Intensive anti-Semitism formed an integral component of the nationalist ideology of the Nazi Party in Germany, which emerged as a major force in the interwar period. It tapped into a cultural anti-Jewish sentiment that preceded the formation of the German state and remained barely beneath the surface during the era of the German Empire or Kaiserreich between 1871 and 1918. During this era, many anti-Jewish barriers were lifted that in turn contributed to Jewish visibility in civil society. This was especially the case in medicine. Jewish participation rose from 3 percent at the start of the nineteenth century to 16 percent at the start of the twentieth century.[2] Not unlike their experiences with the civil service and the military, in the medical faculties as well German Jews faced obstacles in joining the ranks of the university elite. A few rose to become associate professors, but the largest number toiled as Privatdozent or unsalaried lecturers.[3] The economic crisis associated with the aftermath of defeat in World War I led to a resurgence of anti-Semitism in the public culture during the Weimar Republic, spanning 1919 to 1933. Jews were denounced as part of an international conspiracy of Communists and bankers. Their removal from national institutions was regarded as essential in purifying the German nation. Even before the passage of the 1935 Nuremberg Laws, which stripped Jews of their rights as citizens, the medical profession closed ranks in participating in the logic of Nazi ideology. In 1933 Jewish doctors were removed from medical panels servicing the national insurance program and replaced by "Aryan" doctors. In 1935 an ordinance prohibited either the full or partial licensing of doctors who were Jewish, and later Nazi authorities forbade Jews from describing themselves as doctors.[4]

With educational and economic horizons in medicine shrinking, German Jews looked abroad. Opportunities on the Continent were limited. Most countries preferred to protect their professions and imposed steep conditions for foreign nationals to practice medicine legally. Medical education was no less challenging. In France and Switzerland, the presence of foreign and native Jews in medical schools occasioned anti-Semitic and xenophobic protests from students.[5] By comparison, Britain presented a more attractive destination, though it is important not to overstate it. Until the 1880s, the total Jewish population in Britain was relatively small, numbering less 100,000 and distributed unevenly throughout the archipelago. As members of a religious minority within a Protestant confessional state, Jews' participation in society was restricted by laws that required an oath to support the Christian faith. Over the course of the nineteenth century, the campaign for Jewish emancipation gathered momentum, leading to the repeal of restrictions on officeholding, membership in parliament, and admissions to Oxford and Cambridge Universities.

The lingering effects of overt and covert anti-Semitism, suppressed the number of Jews in medicine in the second half of the nineteenth century. There were an estimated twenty-eight Jewish doctors in Britain at midcentury. By the turn of the twentieth century, their numbers had easily doubled.

Scottish institutions proved to be far more open than their English counterparts. The democratic ideal of higher education drew English- and Scottish-born Jews, Jewish colonists from British South Africa and Jamaica, and American Jews to Scottish universities.[6] This tradition, the opportunity associated with medicine, and the growth in the size of the Anglo-Jewish community due in large part to eastern European migration all contributed to greater Jewish participation in medicine by World War I. Medical centers in London, Leeds, and Manchester, with larger Jewish communities than Scottish cities, admitted a growing number of British Jews. But Glasgow and Edinburgh had surpassed them by the 1930s. The number of Jewish medical students grew from eighteen in 1919 to thirty-two in 1924, reaching fifty-one by 1939.[7]

In contrast to other countries, Britain possessed a relatively transparent system for entry into the medical market. Requalification opened up the possibility of practice in the United Kingdom and in reciprocating dominions in the Commonwealth as well in as Italy and Japan. The nonuniversity licensing bodies or the royal professional colleges administered this route independently of the GMC, though the diplomas were registrable. These institutions functioned as examining bodies at prescribed points in the medical education of students over a five-year period. The milestones generally consisted of examinations on medical knowledge in year 2 or 3 and a final professional examination after at least one year of clinical experience in year 4 or 5. While requalification offered a route to the register, it was by no means assured. Eligibility was subject to the discretion of the examining body. By contrast, medical graduates or doctors from reciprocating countries were spared this uncertainty because the GMC had already recognized the qualification. Both medical students and doctors from nonreciprocating countries had to present evidence to satisfy eligibility conditions for each milestone examination or otherwise be required to satisfy them in the United Kingdom.

Requalification was complicated by the legal status of alien immigrants. British policy had discouraged settlement among those immigrants, particularly eastern European Jews who fled pogroms in Russia. The 1905 Aliens Act provided for port controls and inspection. These controls checked the flow of applicants for immigration. The eruption of anti-Jewish persecution in Russia and Poland during the World War I era spurred significant movements of people from eastern to western Europe. The Aliens Act was replaced by legislation that gave the Home Office broad powers to restrict immigration and to deport illegal immigrants. While the assessment of a potential immigrant's financial means was not a condition of entry, this changed in 1919. Thereafter, immigrants were not only subjected to a means test but also lost the right to appeal any "refusal to land" decision. Port immigration personnel possessed wide discretion to limit the length of stay and to prohibit employment as conditions of entry. Although an estimated 120,000 to 150,000 immigrant Jews settled in Britain between 1881 and 1914, these measures were designed to discourage long-term settlement. By the time German Jews began to arrive in significant numbers beginning in 1933, "Britain," as Louise London has written, "no longer was a country of immigration. Strict controls on alien immigrants were now the rule. Entry leading to permanent settlement was restricted to two categories of foreigners only: those whose presence offered some benefit to the country or the people with strong personal or compassionate grounds."[8]

Alarmed by the persecution in central Europe, British Jews led the response to the refugee crisis while the government made accommodations where possible. Influential members of the Anglo-Jewish community lobbied the government to adjust the conditions for entry to Britain. Neville Laski (president of the Board of Deputies of British Jews), Otto Schiff (a merchant banker and president of the Jews' Temporary Shelter), Leonard Montefiore (president of the Anglo-Jewish Association), and Lionel Cohen (a barrister and chairman of the Board of Deputies' Law, Parliamentary, and General Purposes Committee) persuaded the government to relax the condition that refugees demonstrate independence and permit Jewish relief organizations, such as the Jews' Temporary Shelter, to guarantee financial assistance and housing. This relaxation was presented as a temporary measure that would involve only a relatively small number of refugees who would reemigrate. To this end, members such as Schiff participated in Home Office discussions regarding the categories and selection of refugees who would be appropriate candidates for admission to Britain.[9] Ultimately, 50 percent of Jewish refugees admitted to Britain were from the professions. This proportion reflected the selection process as well as the existence of advocacy organizations such as Academic Assistance Council (later known as the Society for the Protection for Science and learning, or SPSL), led by prominent non-Jewish Britons such as the London School of Economics director Sir William Beveridge. Among all occupational groups, dentists and medical professionals accounted for the largest number of professionals among Jewish refugees in 1933. However, admission to Britain was no guarantee of the right to practice medicine.[10]

As early as 1932, nonuniversity licensing bodies were skeptical about making special provisions for refugees with medical training. In a meeting with Home Secretary Sir John Gilmour, representatives of the leading English medical bodies were blunt. As for the potential contributions of German doctors to British medicine and science, Lord Lawson, the president of the Royal College of Physicians, volunteered that "the number that could be usefully absorbed or teach us anything could be counted on the fingers of one hand." The president of the Royal College of Surgeons Sir Holbert Waring alluded to the "annoyance of authorities" when Jewish students at

Edinburgh left for the United States for presumably better career opportunities after completing their training.[11] The reluctance of the elite of institutional British medicine to accept Jewish students was reinforced by the reluctance exhibited by organized medicine. The BMA urged school deans to use their discretion over admission to require final professional examinations and to extend the minimum period of clinical experience from one to three years. Appealing to a narrow definition of British medicine, the association justified this adjustment in familiar terms: concern about potentially treating foreign nationals preferentially over domestic medical students and a commitment to ensuring public safety. In 1934 the medical bodies, with the exception of the Scottish Conjoint Board, agreed to increase the minimum length of required clinical experience to three years.[12]

The boundaries of British medicine were drawn even more tightly in the Commonwealth. In 1934 the Medical Council of South Africa proposed an amendment to local regulations that extended the minimum length of time of professional study to three years in the country in which the diploma was awarded. While prolonging the period of residency was consistent with the policy of all but one of the British-based licensing bodies, local medical authorities were at the time concerned that the terms of reciprocity might be breached. If adopted, the holders of qualifications of the Scottish Conjoint Board—a scheduled licensing body in the United Kingdom—would not be entitled to local registration in South Africa. The South African medical council therefore sought advice on whether the amendment "would be regarded as infringing their 'just' privileges of doctors registered in the United Kingdom." The concern proved to be unwarranted. In a memo to the Lord President Sir Maurice Hankey, E. C. E. Leadbitter reported no objections were likely to be raised by the council. In fact, King, a representative from the Scottish board, assured Leadbitter of no serious protest from his board.[13]

Between 1933 and 1935, some 180 German doctors requalified in the United Kingdom. Before Britain entered into the war in early September 1939, another one hundred refugees (fifty from Austria and fifty from Czechoslovakia) were permitted to requalify.[14] This latter cohort, like other Jews, fled in the wake of the German territorial aggrandizement in Austria and Czechoslovakia and intensified attacks on the minority Jewish communities. In a significant precedent, however, even after requalifying, this group's right to practice in the United Kingdom was not unrestricted. Deferring to the profession's concern about glutting the metropolitan market, the Home Office restricted the first cohort of medical refugees to areas outside of London. Those who were permitted to requalify later were prohibited from practicing in the United Kingdom altogether. Their immigration status as aliens preempted the rights of doctors on the register. As aliens, employment, no less than settlement, was a privilege, not a right, overseen by the

Home Office. There was little objection from the organized medical profession. BMA representatives on the Home Office Medical Advisory Committee pushed for limiting the numbers of refugees to be qualified and for restrictions on their rights of practice. Even over the decision of the government to accommodate a larger number of refugees for admission, the committee justified narrow portals to medical practice to privilege British-born and -qualified medical graduates. These views were not those of the association alone. Other representatives of the British medical establishment were on the committee, including the nonuniversity licensing bodies and the GMC.[15]

The Limitations of Medical Reciprocity: Jewish Doctors in Italy and the GMC

In comparison to Germany, Italy was a safe harbor—at least for a few years. For German Jewish doctors and medical students, there were fewer obstacles to admission to the royal universities.[16] Based on the 1924 agreement between Italy and the United Kingdom, recipients of Italian medical degrees were entitled to registration in Britain and elsewhere in reciprocating dominions. In light of the deteriorating situation in Germany and Britain's reluctance to admit Jewish refugees in general and foreign doctors in particular, GMC registrar Michael Helestine was anxious to learn more about the conditions for foreign Jewish medical students and doctors in Italy. The assurances of the Italian Embassy were contradicted by the inquiries from foreign doctors in Italy. Subsequently, Helestine reminded the Privy Council of Britain's involvement under the reciprocity agreement. "From our point of view, as you know, the matter is important not only because we may in the not too distant future be required to register an unknown number of German Jews with Italian refugees on the Foreign List of the Register, but also because under the agreement of 1925, such registration carries with it the right to practice in the British Dominions and Colonies where medical reciprocity exists, subject, I think, to any local law in a Dominion which may restrict the completeness of reciprocity."[17]

Helestine's concern was prescient. Until 1938 Italy had not adopted explicit anti-Jewish policies even though Mussolini had forged an alliance with Germany. In 1936 he entered into the Berlin-Rome Axis with Hitler, which outlined a future realignment of power in Europe. Anti-Communism formed a key component, especially after the outbreak of the Spanish Civil War. The Anti-Comintern Pact, which was also signed by Japan, underscored this budding relationship. The status for Italian and non-Italian Jews became insecure as Italy was remade in the image of fascism. Both state-sponsored and -endorsed anti-Semitism in the mass media grew, defining Jews as inherently suspect.[18] Within the profession, the provincial Ordini dei Medici was replaced by the Fashistian Medical Syndicate.[19] In March 1935 a royal decree prohibited all non-Italians from practicing medicine. This decree targeted German Jewish refugees. It permitted them to study and receive qualifications but not to settle and practice in Italy. The decree also closed off Italy's East African Empire.[20] The official acts of anti-Semitism culminated in the 1938 decree. This decree altered the legal and social standing of Italian Jews. It narrowly defined Italian citizenship to exclude Jews. Any Jewish persons who obtained their citizenship after 1919 were now deemed noncitizens. Even Jews who were citizens were subjected to discriminatory legislation, including the loss of public titles and positions, including those in the civil service and universities. Combined with the 1935 decree that prohibited non-Italians from practicing medicine, the 1938 decree made it a crime for all non-Italian Jews to practice medicine. The effect was predictable: foreign Jewish doctors looked outside the borders of Italy.[21]

For Helestine, these decrees implicated the GMC in anti-Semitic policies. They imperiled Jewish doctors who qualified in Italy and sought to take advantage of admission to the register under the terms of reciprocity between Italy and Britain. But section 17 of the Medical Act required that the applicants for registration in the United Kingdom possess a recognized degree that legally entitled them to practice medicine in the country that granted the primary qualification. Admitting such foreign-trained doctors to the register would be a technical violation of part 2 of the Medical Act. Unless the Anglo-Italian treaty was amended, the status quo effectively endorsed the discriminatory purpose of the decree. Helestine sought clarification about the status of the treaty with the Foreign Office.[22]

The Foreign Office was indifferent to foreign and native Jewish doctors in Italy. Intervening on behalf of foreign doctors in Italy risked upsetting delicate diplomatic relations at a time when an Italian-German alliance was becoming more problematic for Britain. It was unlikely that support existed within the British medical profession for amending the treaty. In light of the reluctance to increase the number of Jewish refugee doctors from Germany and Austria, the Foreign Office announced itself satisfied with the status quo. The legal advisor to the Foreign Office, John Samos, spelled out Britain's understanding of the scope of the treaty. If anything, Britain's diplomatic relationship with Italy appeared to minimize the effects. Samos writes: "I am to state that, as far as Lord Halifax is aware, there are no Jewish doctors of British nationality at present resident in Italy. Moreover the Italian authorities have been given wide discretion to grant exemption from the application of the anti-Jewish legislation in individual cases. In fact it does not appear that any British subjects have as yet been required to leave Italy by reason of their Jewish connexion or that any will be compelled to do so." While Samos conceded that Jews could be forced to leave under the decree, he noted that the discretion of the authorities "has been exercised in favor of those Jews of British nationality who wish to remain in Italy."[23]

Even in the Commonwealth, the council's authority had become significantly attenuated. Following a Privy Council law opinion concerning legislation in New Zealand in 1924 that barred Italian doctors on the foreign list of the British register from local registration, the capacity of the GMC to use the register to reconcile the national and imperial boundaries of medicine was reduced. This was made all the more clear as medically trained refugees confronted hurdles and barriers in the Commonwealth. South Africa was not the only Commonwealth country to limit, if not prevent, medically trained refugees from entering into practice. Like South Africa, states in the federated commonwealth of Australia began to restrict access, citing the need to protect the economic interests of the indigenous profession. At the request of the Victoria medical board, the state legislature in 1938 amended registration regulations. Under the new law, foreign doctors would have to complete a minimum of five years of study in the state or in the reciprocating country that awarded the qualifications.[24] Other states adopted similar legislation. In New South Wales foreign graduates were required to sit for the fourth, fifth, and final professional examinations as prescribed by Sydney University, provided that they were from a reciprocating jurisdiction.[25] Up until 1938, New Zealand was generous in its accommodation by comparison. Its medical council not only directed refugees with medical training to complete a three-year course at Otago University as a condition of local registration, but also recognized the qualifications of doctors who obtained Scottish certificates. In 1939, however, its portals shrank. The council began capping the annual number of refugees with medical degrees to be admitted and also issued notices that disconnected entry to the Dominion from the right to practice medicine.[26]

The GMC responded to these changes in much the same way it had in the recent past: after the fact. Neither state medical authorities nor Commonwealth representatives consulted the GMC in advance of legislation. Short of recommending the revocation of reciprocity to the Privy Council, the GMC could only seek clarification or raise concerns about compliance infractions in hopes of persuading local authorities to make adjustments. Preferring the broadest scope for British medicine, the GMC in practice recommended revocation only after exhausting consultation with reciprocating countries or territories. But the matter was not simply or strictly about compliance. The GMC's own acceptance of unequal treatment of refugees created the appearance of a double standard. While it was appropriate to limit or even to prohibit refugee doctors on the register from practice in the United Kingdom, it apparently was not for other medical authorities in the Commonwealth.

It is likely for these reasons that GMC president Norman Walker chose his language carefully when discussing the matter in public. In his presidential address during the summer session, he resisted asserting a metropolitan response to the refugee crisis, deferring instead to local authorities as most competent to make determinations. Walker acknowledged that "medical registration is a complex problem on which different opinions are inevitably and legitimately held in different quarters of the globe."[27] He conceded also that local decisions may have been a product of the "the strain of urgent demands for registration from quarters perhaps un-welcomed." At the same time, Walker was critical of the unilateral nature of these decisions, partly because of their impact on Jewish refugee doctors and partly because of the effect on the credibility of the GMC. Although the GMC was charged with overseeing part 2 of the Medical Act, medical authorities were not required to consult with the registrar or the president before amending or adopting new medical regulations. In the absence of regular communication and consultation, Walker pointed out that the council was reduced to learning in the press about new laws that might have a bearing on the rights of doctors on the register.[28] Later, Walker appealed directly to local medical authorities in Victoria and New South Wales.[29] Seeking to mitigate overcrowding anxieties, he noted that less than a dozen doctors would need to be accommodated. Once admitted to the register, they would also be entitled to practice in other reciprocating countries. Walker added that the five-year condition of practice in either Britain or the receiving country was not strictly in line with the reciprocity agreements. At the same time, he neglected to mention that their immigration status significantly limited the place and duration of the practice of medicine in the United Kingdom.[30] Walker's efforts yielded no results: neither Victoria nor New South Wales changed its regulations.

Managing British Medicine during World War: The Creation of the Temporary Register

Once Britain entered the war, British medicine opened again. As in World War I, the recruitment of university-age men and medical practitioners for military service diminished the supply of future medical school entrants and reduced the effective strength of the medical profession. Policy makers understood the value of opening the register. Foreign doctors expanded the personnel capacity of the domestic profession and underscored the political ties between the United Kingdom and allied and neutral countries. Within the first year, the War Cabinet adopted Defense Regulation 32 B, which empowered the GMC to add to the British register a doctor who is "by law entitled to practice medicine, surgery and midwifery" in a given British territory, by the order of the health secretary. This regulation was closely followed by The Medical (Temporary Registration) Order of 1940, which permitted "for the duration of the present emergency only" the registration of "British subjects and American citizens holding medical diplomas granted in Canada and the United States and not normally registrable in the United Kingdom."[31] Private practice was strictly prohibited. The selection of these countries was no accident. Both US president Franklin Roosevelt and Canadian prime minister William Lyon MacKenzie King were sympathetic to Britain at this early stage in the war when public opinion in each country was against or at least divided about joining the war effort. Quite apart from the political and propaganda benefits, the terms of this order opened the Emergency Medical Service to American and Canadian doctors, thereby freeing up British doctors for military service.[32]

This order represented a significant development for the GMC. It added a third route to the register for overseas-trained doctors.[33] The geographical scale of British medicine now expanded to include all of North America. So too did the authority of the council. In interpreting the order, the council alone recognized diplomas for purposes of registration and confirmed that the overseas practitioners were entitled by law to practice medicine. This discretionary power had been long sought by the council. Each previous attempt to amend the Medical Act along these lines had been defeated on grounds that foreign graduates would be admitted to the medical register on far more favorable terms than British graduates while placing the British public at risk. Further, the order was noteworthy because the medical schools and colleges in either country were not subject to inspection. In exchange for securing the cooperation of American and Canadian doctors, the council accepted the qualifications as providing sufficient evidence of the effective practice of medicine in the United Kingdom. Oversight of the Medical Council of Canada for medical education in the Dominion, together with provincial bodies managing local licensing, minimized the risk of admitting doctors with dubious qualifications to the register. Even in the case of the United States, the GMC relied on the experience of non-university licensing bodies for Americans who had requalified as well as the judgments of both the American Medical Association and National Board of Medical Examiners in the United States.

As much as the order was designed to allow for an orderly admission to the register for medical graduates from North America, pressure grew for further expansion. Before and during the spring of 1940, German armies occupied Poland, the Netherlands and France, among other countries. French and Dutch refugees in Britain included civilian and military medical personnel. Their numbers added to those from Poland and Czechoslovakia. The order established a precedent for further amendment. In June 1940, Michiels van Verduynen of the Netherlands legation sought permission to permit Dutch doctors to practice among nationals in a letter to Foreign Secretary Viscount Halifax.[34]

In response to van Verduynen's request, GMC registrar Helestine outlined two options available to the Privy Council. As professionals from a nonreciprocating country, doctors from the Netherlands could requalify in either the United Kingdom or Ireland while obtaining a work permit from the Home Office under the Aliens Reconstruction Act; or, alternatively, the government could modify the temporary registration order to include the Netherlands. In a confidential memo, Helestine pointed out that requalification was impractical, given the mandatory five-year period of study. Work permits were equally problematic, but for different reasons. In this case, the status of these doctors from the Netherlands as nonregistered would remain unchanged in the eyes of the GMC. Registered doctors were prohibited from engaging nonregistered doctors to cover for them during temporary absences. Although the council was prepared to look the other way, it would have to act if charges of misconduct were raised.[35] Temporary registration was the most direct route for qualifying doctors from an eligible country, provided that the order was amended. This option however involved a trade-off, namely accommodating the needs of an ally without "first hand knowledge of the standard of qualifications granted in the Netherlands." Helestine was confident that the council would be able to obtain this knowledge through the Netherlands legation, through the institutional experience of the nonlicensing bodies in England and Scotland, and through interviews with candidates whose qualifications were awarded in the Netherlands.[36]

In January 1941, the government put into effect an amended order for temporary registration. The order empowered the council to admit to the foreign list of the temporary register nationals "now in this country—the majority of them refugees—who hold diplomas granted in foreign countries, other than America." The eligible doctors reflected the disruption caused by the war, and included those "(a) who hold, or have been selected for, medical commissions in the Armed Forces of the Crown or in an allied or Associated Force; (b) who are employed or have been selected for employment as medical officers in hospitals, institution or service (not involving medical attendance on patients in their own homes) for the time being approved by the Minister for the purpose of the Order."[37] The application of the order included a far larger number of countries than the original request from the Netherlands. Eligible countries now included allied and occupied countries France, Belgium, Germany, the Netherlands, Norway, Czechoslovakia, Italy, and Poland as well as the dominions, the colonies within the Commonwealth and mandated territories. Under this order and its predecessor, some 868 practitioners were registered: 96 from the British Empire and 772 from foreign countries.[38]

While this amended order addressed new developments in the war, its operation highlighted the limitations of the register in mediating British medicine in the world. Even though the register increased by ten allied and enemy countries, section 17 of the Medical Act of 1886 complicated access. Under this section, the council was obligated to confirm that its qualifications entitled foreign doctors to practice medicine in the country where they qualified. This relationship between medicine and state assumed that credentialed doctors enjoyed equal standing within and among states. By abiding by section 17, the council policed the boundaries of British medicine and promoted medicine as a liberal profession. But its experience with displaced doctors and medical refugees exposed the limitations of the register. Jews in Germany, Austria, and Italy who were stripped of their legal rights to practice medicine—even though they possessed qualifications that entitled non-Jews to practice—could not satisfy section 17. By abiding by the legal title provision, the council became complicit in extending prewar anti-Jewish laws to the United Kingdom.[39]

Wartime conditions were also not optimal for establishing legal title to practice for displaced doctors. The movement of people from countries where they qualified and the international character of armies made ascertaining legal title based on the location of qualification or territory of commission difficult, if not impossible.[40] While the amended order was flexible enough to accommodate these situations, it placed a substantial administrative burden on the GMC. Lack of experience with the universities and professional bodies in eligible countries stretched the council's informational resources and institutional memory. The nonuniversity licensing bodies in the United Kingdom, to be sure, afforded assistance based on their evaluation of the qualifications from nonreciprocating countries. Provisional registration permitted doctors to practice while the council verified their credentials. Still, even the GMC conceded that its temporary registration decisions were based on "incomplete knowledge."[41]

The order was a mixed blessing for employers and not least for displaced doctors and medically trained refugees. Outside of a military commission, employment was a prerequisite for temporary registration and limited to three categories: local authority hospitals, institutions, and clinics; institutions associated with the Emergency Medical Service; and ship surgeons on British vessels. The machinery for work permits was designed to assess the character, potential threat to public safety, and skills of each candidate. The Central Medical War Committee, which advised the government on staffing needs, processed applications on behalf of candidates. The Home Office and the Aliens War Service Department reviewed applications on a case-by-case basis. Once the candidate was approved, the employer was permitted to appoint the doctor. The machinery, which sought to protect the public and the economic interests of British doctors, was criticized as insufficient by local authorities who were under intense pressure to address staffing deficiencies at a time when British medical graduates were in short supply. The conditions of employment not only complicated the deployment of these doctors but also reminded them of their contingent and conditional presence within the social landscape of British medicine. According to a Ministry of Health circular, in the event of an invasion or serious military situation, registered foreign doctors from enemy countries were subject to removal from designated or military areas as deemed necessary by military authorities. Within the hospital, local authorities were advised to limit alien doctors to 10 percent of the medical and nursing staff of hospitals with less than one hundred beds and 20 percent of hospitals with more than one hundred. Whenever possible, they were to be employed "in wards where British doctors and nurses" were engaged. In the wards dedicated to military service personnel, "aliens must not be employed."[42]

These defects in the regulation and management of foreign doctors spurred additional calls for amending the order. For the Foreign Office, the register functioned as a political and propagandistic tool while at the same time providing access to medical labor for staffing British hospitals. In early 1941, R. A. Gallop of the South American Department suggested adding to the North American and European regional coverage of the 1940 order. In a letter to A. W. Neville of the Ministry of Health, Gallop described the advantages of including Central and South American countries: "We think that a most valuable political and propaganda effect might be obtained by enrolling suitable volunteers from neutral countries. Conversely, a sense of disappointment and frustration will be engendered if we continue to cold shoulder our neutral well wishers without a clear and convincing explanation of why we do not want their help."[43] The ministry was open to expansion, particularly to neutral countries like Spain and newly allied countries like Yugoslavia and the Duchy of Luxemburg. At the same time, the English-language competency of doctors was raised as a concern about doctors from South America. A condition of registration would require "any such doctors to be classifiable as English speaking, that is to say they would have to have sufficient knowledge of the language to be able to carry on their profession with colleagues and patients who speak no other language."[44]

This language concern did not complicate the Foreign Office rationale for expansion. It had already added all of North America. "The propaganda point raised in Gallop's letter to the Chief Medical Officer Neville is one which applies to American countries, where, as he explained, we attach considerable importance to it," wrote A. W. G. Randall.[45] "So far as European countries are concerned we are in general guided by utilitarian considerations." These considerations referred to the goal of harnessing even more allied and neutral countries to the war effort when Britain remained the last hope for Europe. Randall floated an ambitious expansion of participating countries beyond those originally contemplated. "Would it perhaps be worth considering taking only one bite at the cherry and including all European countries? This would involve, apart from the amendment of the reference to the Netherlands and the addition of Luxemburg, mention of Spain, Portugal, Sweden, Finland, Denmark, Estonia, Latvia, Lithuania, Romania, Hungary, Bulgaria and Yugoslavia." He was equally expansive about applying the regulation to American countries. "We should certainly wish it to be all or none. They are, of course, the United States, Mexico, Honduras, Salvador, Nicaragua, Costa Rica, Panama, Haiti, the Dominican Republic, Colombia, Venezuela, Brazil, Paraguay, Argentina, and Chile."[46]

From the summer through the fall, the health ministry officials consulted with the GMC along with other government offices and statutory bodies involved in the management of foreign doctors. The suggested changes included removing the phrase "by law entitled to practice" from Defense Regulation 32B, expanding the number of countries eligible for temporary registration, and abolishing employment as a precondition of temporary registration in the Medical Regulation Order. Collectively, these and other changes would broaden access to the register in the service of the political, propagandistic, and personnel needs of the war effort. For the council, these benefits were not without problems. If anything, they highlighted the tension between the internationalization of the war effort and the job of regulating the boundaries of British medicine. As conveyed in Helestine's memo, the council was frustrated with the limited means to ascertain legal title.[47] Recognizing the difficulty of checking qualifications of all foreign-trained temporarily registered medical personnel, the council, not surprisingly, called for the revocation of section 17.

Its recent experience with assessing the qualifications of candidates from the countries covered by the amended 1940 order added to the council's skepticism about its capacity to guarantee even a minimum standard of competence from a new, much larger pool of candidates. In that case, interviews with candidates had helped to supplement knowledge about qualifications granted in the countries covered by the order as well as a few exceptional cases from countries not covered, such as Estonia, Russia, Spain, and Switzerland, and had also provided the council with confidence that public safety would not be jeopardized. However, Helestine doubted that the council could give such assurance for the number of countries contemplated under the proposed order. In the absence of safeguards, such as an interview and selection for an appointment in the United Kingdom, the order created the risk of flooding the medical market with foreign doctors of unknown competence and motivation.[48]

The council opposed revoking the employment requirement as a condition of temporary registration for medical refugees. It was the only safeguard for evaluating the professional experience and competence of foreign doctors once the council recognized their diploma.[49] The employment interview served as a means to regulate access to British medicine. Far from being within the competency of the council, Helestine regarded the interview as appropriate, if not a duty, for members of the staff of British hospitals. Qualified and registered in the United Kingdom, these doctors were equipped to assess the professional training and experience of candidates. The employment interview had many functions, not least the determination of competency. Born and bred in the United Kingdom, British doctors also protected the safety and security of the public from imposters. Helestine noted that the council was responsible for the prevention of and investigation into medical identity theft. By contrast, a searching interview was more likely than not to expose contradictions in candidates' accounts of their training and country of birth. Exposure ensured not only the integrity of the register and credibility of hospitals, but also the expulsion of undesirables from the country.[50]

Whatever the political gains that might be obtained by relaxing access to the register, Helestine warned of substantial political consequences in and outside of the government. Temporary registration implicated other departments of state. It conferred on foreign doctors the right to prescribe medication. The supervision of the Dangerous Drugs Act was the responsibility of the Home Office, which also supervised immigration. Helestine anticipated departmental resistance by framing the presumed threat of foreign doctors in racially coded terms, specifically by mentioning nonwhite countries or regions that were Muslim and Catholic: "Are the Home Office satisfied that the authorization of an unknown number of doctors from such territories as Egypt, Turkey, and those of South America may not, if the employment of the doctors is not restricted to approved hospitals or other institutions or services, and no provision is made for interview of the foreign practitioners by British doctors, lead to abuse of the Dangerous Drugs Acts by the doctors and to their British patients?"

Liberal terms of entry would likely provoke the Ministry of Health and the BMA. Helestine noted that doctors admitted to the temporary register would be eligible to treat patients covered under the National Insurance Scheme. The scheme—administered by the ministry—covered members of the skilled working classes. To be sure, the right to engage in insurance practice would free up indigenous doctors to serve in the armed forces. But as Helestine insinuated, this right opened the government to criticism for enabling different standards of care for working-class communities; similarly, the presence of foreign doctors replacing British doctors who were making sacrifices on behalf of the nation also made the government vulnerable to criticism. While this would be a temporary measure, the potential existed for foreign doctors to remain in Britain after the end of the war. "Professional organizations of British doctors (of which the Council are not one) will presumably not be slow to point that the more generously the

Register is opened to temporary registration, the stronger is the vested interest in favor of converting temporary registration in to permanent registration,"[51] Helestine commented.

Although the council clearly had serious reservations about the proposals, they did not close out a compromise, particularly about recognizing foreign diplomas. Council president H. L. Eason and Helestine continued their conversation with the ministry. Given the admittedly incomplete knowledge about the qualification process in designated countries, the adoption of the order as proposed might not produce the political benefits hoped for, but rather the opposite. Domestically, registering doctors whose training was deemed to be not equivalent to that of those in the United Kingdom created the potential for far-reaching consequences in the event of a single adverse experience with a foreign doctor. Even if the draft order was modified to include a selective listing of countries, it "might give offense internationally." As a compromise solution, Easom proposed replacing the list of countries in which the order was to be applied with the phrase "any foreign country." In summarizing the costs and benefits, Beckett found this compromise workable: "Theoretically, this is still open to the objection that a doctor from a country with a low standard of medical training could claim to be considered, but he is not in such a strong position as he would be if his country were specifically named by the Order."[52]

In September, the amended order was adopted by the War Cabinet. Like its predecessors, it reflected a compromise between wartime needs and the regulation of British medicine. Temporary registration was open to all eligible candidates. Candidates within the territorial jurisdiction of the United Kingdom had to be legally entitled to practice medicine, surgery, and midwifery while all others had to hold either "a medical qualification granted in any such place, or has passed the examination necessary to obtain such diploma."[53] The employment condition for medical refugees was retained. The prohibition on private practice was slightly relaxed. Those on the temporary register could be employed as assistants to practitioners in existing partnership practices. The amended order did not dilute the authority of the GMC but increased it. Previously, its discretion to recognize qualifications was confined to the United States and Canada and later expanded to include allied and neutral countries for the most part in western Europe. The council was now empowered to evaluate medical qualifications from virtually anywhere in the world for purposes of temporary registration.

Legacies of the War: Temporary Registration and the Power to Register Foreign Doctors, 1945–48

The passage of the amended order took place two months before a major development in the war: the attack on the military installation at Pearl

Harbor in the US territory of Hawaii on December 7 by the imperial government of Japan. This attack broadened the nature of the conflict. The declaration of war by the United States and United Kingdom against Japan was matched three days later by that of Germany and Italy against the United States. Britain's declaration of war in 1939 against the Axis Powers effectively terminated their reciprocal relationships with Italy and Japan. The 1942 amended order more than compensated for the loss of these two countries. Temporary registration was open to any eligible medical profession from anywhere in the world, including allied, neutral, and enemy countries. Between 1943 and 1945, the numbers on the foreign list grew, comprising a broad spectrum of countries from western and eastern Europe to North, South, and Central America.

In retrospect, the internationalization of the register would have been inconceivable prior to the outbreak of war, given the resistance of organized medicine and the medical establishment to the admission of medically trained refugees. The combined effect of the political and personnel needs of Britain created a compelling environment for admitting more overseas-trained doctors. Crucial to this shift was an integrated set of conditions for registration that preserved the economic and social boundaries of British medicine while addressing the expanding health care needs of a nation engaged in total war. These conditions prescribed the duration of registration, limited the types of employment, and restricted private practice. Underlying these conditions was the assumption that foreign doctors would leave and return to their homelands. But as the war came to a close, the temporality of registration and growing Soviet influence in Poland and elsewhere complicated the return to prewar conditions of British medicine.

The repatriation of "stateless" people became for all practical purposes impossible and led to a far more permissive basis for the naturalization of refugees, including alien doctors. In signaling its shift in policy in 1946, the Home Office in a letter to the BMA laid out the case for permitting alien doctors to continue to practice in Britain. Although foreign born, their service during the war and their familiarity with "the usages and standards of the British medical profession" underscored a shared appreciation of British medicine. Their numbers were small and it was expected that the postwar production of future British doctors would assure the national character of the profession. Spurring this shift was the scheduled termination of temporary registration in February 1946 as provided for in the Emergency Laws (Transitional Provisions) Act. The act abolished temporary registration as a category and scheduled the termination of the rights to practice of those on the list by the end of 1947. While the register did close at this time to new entrants, nearly 3,500 foreign doctors were already in Britain. After the departure of Americans and Canadians, some 1,500 to 2,000 doctors from Germany, Austria, Poland, and Czechoslovakia would be subject to the conditions of the act.[54]

Any change in the registration status of foreign doctors involved the GMC, particularly its power to admit foreign doctors to the register. The Defense Regulation 32B extended this authority for the duration of the war. Over this period, the council obtained experience in regulating the admission of foreign-trained doctors. The various sources of information about qualifications plus employment-related safeguards provided a method for ensuring that foreign and colonial doctors possessed a minimum standard of professional competence to practice medicine in the United Kingdom and its territories and among personnel in the armed forces. As the termination of temporary registration loomed, in early 1947 the government drafted legislation to accommodate affected foreign doctors. The provisions of the draft legislation approximated the conditions for temporary registration during the war. First, residency in the United Kingdom and military service were limiting conditions. The former restricted eligibility to medically trained refugees and displaced doctors who relocated to Britain. The latter referred to those who held commissions in the armed forces. Second, those doctors who were temporarily registered had only to furnish proof of rendering satisfactory service in a designated clinical position—in a hospital or private practice setting—to satisfy the council's condition of competency. Commissioned medical officers had to possess a medical qualification.[55]

The council not only supported the expansion of its authority to admit foreign doctors to the register, but also called for establishing temporary registration as a new category of registration. If the experience of the war had taught any lesson, it was the mobility of medical labor. Reciprocity and requalification had proven to be insufficiently flexible. Temporary registration, by contrast, expanded access to labor as well as support for the British war effort without compromising the statutory responsibility of the GMC. Safeguards—such as prescribed duration, prohibited career appointments, and restricted private practice—preserved the social and economic integrity of British medicine. In the postwar period as during the war, temporary registration would enable Britain to manage access to national medicine while engaging with the world more instrumentally.

Temporary registration would also enable Britain to project its impact more widely by training the world's doctors. Drawing on prewar and wartime frustrations, Helestine drew attention to the "'anomolous [*sic*] position' of distinguished medical and surgical visitors to this country, who could not obtain even the most transitory form of medical registration, while demonstrating their methods in a hospital such as Guy's."[56] Helestine stressed "a need for some form of registration to be available for doctors coming to this country to continue their professional education in temporary appointments in Hospitals (normally in Teaching Hospitals)." This aspect of temporary registration built on the historical relationship between the GMC and the empire and Commonwealth in which metropolitan university and nonuniversity licensing bodies recognized colonial equivalents to satisfy conditions to sit for the staggered professional examinations. These included the university general education degree or certificate and hospital experience. The ensuing colonial and metropolitan relationships laid the foundation for the GMC recognition of diplomas for admission to the register from colonies or territories that reciprocated with the United Kingdom.[57]

While registration permitted colonial and foreign medical graduates to seek advanced training and experience in an approved hospital or clinical setting, medical specialties were largely closed off. The informal nature of the social production of hospital-based specialists privileged doctors who qualified in the United Kingdom. Consultants occupied the peak of the staffing hierarchy. In this position, they served as gatekeepers. Appointments and associated opportunities for clinical experience were subject to the informal networks and approval of elite practitioners. Access to such professional networks privileged British medical graduates more so than colonial or foreign graduates. Temporary registration would not affect the hierarchy of power within the hospital, but rather normalize the continuing professional education of foreign and colonial medical graduates.

This rationale echoed a larger push to incorporate hospital-based training as a formal dimension of continuing medical education. Advocates for the reform of medical education called for change in response to the growth of medical knowledge and the expanded duties of the practitioner. Continuing postgraduate training was essential, not optional. Adding to an overcrowded medical school curriculum was not the answer. Instead, they argued for mandating yearlong clinical instruction under the supervision of a senior hospital staff doctor before medical graduates were admitted to the register. This was a major recommendation of the 1944 *Report by the Inter-Departmental Committee on Medical Schools*, chaired by Sir William Goodenough. The committee, like the parallel committee that had produced the blueprint for the National Health Service two years earlier, was appointed by the wartime government with a specific charge: to plan for the postwar society. Each medical graduate would complete a rotation through the main hospital departments—medical, surgical, and midwifery—under the supervision of senior members of the staff. The effect of this recommendation would be far-reaching. It would expand the number of hospitals engaged in training while ensuring that all doctors were equipped to practice medicine. Within the hospital, doctors from Britain and the rest of the world would advance British medicine while serving the British public.

The government incorporated temporary registration into the 1948 Medical Practitioners and Pharmacists Act. The act broadened the power of the council to register foreign and colonial doctors, specifically those who were on the temporary register under the Defense Regulation 32B or the Polish Resettlement Act, who served in the British armed forces (including

Indian forces and Burma forces) and who "were permitted to enter the United Kingdom through circumstances attributable to the war."[58] The provision for registration was a reward to foreign and Commonwealth doctors who contributed to the war effort. But the period of eligibility was finite: six months for doctors in category 1 and twelve months for those in categories 2 and 3. At the same time, this restriction was designed to prevent others from exploiting the opportunity while protecting the social and economic composition of British medicine. A similar safeguard was the clause relating to temporary registration. Applicants were required to satisfy the "council that he is or intends to be in the United Kingdom temporarily."[59] This declaration reinforced the conditional nature of the presence of foreign and Commonwealth doctors in the United Kingdom. It discouraged settlement by prohibiting the practice of medicine outside of the constraints of temporary registration.

Conclusion

The passage of the 1948 Act certainly reflected novel conditions associated with the end of World War II. In truth, it marked continuity as much as change. Until 1926, admission to the register entitled all doctors—foreign and colonial alike—to equitable treatment. But in accepting the right of authorities in the dominions to selectively admit only doctors who qualified in the United Kingdom, the Privy Council and the GMC endorsed a precedent for differential treatment. Between 1933 and 1938 Jewish refugee doctors, who were admitted to the register after qualifying in the United Kingdom, were among the first to experience this change. Their statelessness raised deep anxieties about their future place within the profession as well as within the society at large. The BMA, the Home Office, and nonuniversity licensing bodies forged a set of practices that were clearly designed to minimize the economic and social impact of Jewish refugee doctors. Rather than being entitled to unrestricted rights, their alien immigration status restricted the place and length of time they could practice. Britain's entry into the war in 1939 did little to change the unequal treatment of alien (Jewish and non-Jewish) doctors. Successive orders, which opened the register to qualified doctors from allied, neutral, and belligerent countries, expanded the supply of doctors for the home and war fronts. These doctors were granted the unrestricted right of practice during the emergency of war. By contrast, alien doctors were admitted to the register only after they secured an appointment in an approved hospital or clinical setting. This involved an assessment of the candidates' professional competency and, indirectly, their command of the English language during an interview with a member of the medical staff of an employing authority. Until 1941 alien doctors, once admitted to the temporary register, were only permitted to practice in a hospital under the supervision of British medical staff. The final order relaxed the prohibition on private practice by permitting alien doctors to serve as locum tenems, or backup doctors, again under the direction of a member of the British medical profession. The 1948 Act formalized what had been a set of practices that was designed to diminish the disruptions associated with the prewar refugee crisis and war itself. Its processes for temporary and full registration facilitated the orderly postwar globalization of the register. In supplementing the supply of domestic medical graduates, overseas doctors—as in the previous wars—enabled Britain to expand its capacity to deliver health care to the nation.

Part Two

Remaking British Medicine

Chapter Five

From Asset to Liability

Overseas Doctors of Color in the United Kingdom, 1955–70

Introduction

The influx of foreign doctors into Britain was unprecedented in the post–World War II era. By 1955, overseas doctors—fully and temporarily registered—in aggregate far exceeded the annual production of domestic medical graduates. Their presence was no accident. The register continued to serve the national interest of Britain and British medicine even as the empire rapidly contracted. Technical assistance in the form of medical training constituted a major component in sustaining relations among member countries, including new Commonwealth countries in Africa and Asia that obtained their independence after the war. In addition to government-sponsored exchanges and training schemes abroad, domestic professional colleges and hospitals participated in the delivery of assistance to sponsored and unsponsored doctors. Indeed, overseas doctors who returned home with professional experience or additional qualifications advanced Britain's postwar vision of itself as a postimperial world power.

Besides buffing its image, technical assistance translated into an enormous transfer of wealth to Britain from donor countries. Indeed, the labor of overseas doctors was indispensable to the National Health Service (NHS). Launched in 1948, the NHS fulfilled a wartime pledge of comprehensive social security for all British citizens as outlined in the 1942 Beveridge report. Organizationally, the NHS consisted of a hospital service and a network of private practices that contracted with the government. But the delivery of medical care was ultimately dependent on a steady supply of doctors, especially in the hospital service. Even after mandating a preregistration yearlong hospital rotation for all medical graduates in 1952, growing use of services exposed the structural imbalance between the demand and supply of medical labor. Here overseas doctors supplemented the domestic profession. By 1960 they accounted for nearly 40 percent of the medical staff in the junior or training grades. In accommodating the training aspirations of overseas doctors, temporary registration afforded hospitals with an elastic supply of doctors to deliver health care to the public. These doctors provided care in underserved urban and rural hospitals. Their conditions of registration ensured that they would be under the supervision of a senior British member of the hospital staff and would not compete with domestic medical graduates who pursued career advancement in the service or practiced medicine privately.

The movement of doctors to Britain benefited British medicine in another crucial way. The one-time registration fee paid by domestic medical graduates had been the main source of revenue for the operations of the GMC since its founding. As the number of new admissions to the register increasingly replaced exits, the council maintained a hand-to-mouth existence. In the face of growing activity in the postwar era together with the pressure of inflation, this hitherto reliable source of revenue proved to be insufficient. It is for this reason that the growing stream of registration fees from overseas doctors proved to be indispensable. Indeed, the fee structure, particularly for temporary registration, imposed a much higher total financial burden on overseas doctors—who had to continually renew their registration status in order to extend their stay—than the one-time fee for which British medical graduates were responsible. Overseas doctors subsidized the GMC while mitigating the financial burden on British doctors to support the very institution mandated by Parliament to regulate the national profession.

At the same time, the globalization of British medicine at home engendered criticism. Far from preserving the fiction of national homogeneity, the register was increasingly portrayed as an instrument that undermined the social integrity of British medicine. The movement of domestic medical graduates out of Britain rendered overseas doctors of color more visible to the public than ever before. Emigration to the "old" Commonwealth and the United States continued a pattern that predated World War II. But critics within and outside of the profession decried this outflow as nothing less than a national crisis brought on by the socialization of medicine. The exit of domestic medical graduates was seen to be not only a transfer of wealth to other countries but also as an indictment of the NHS. This depletion discourse racialized the presence of overseas doctors in Britain and their place in British medicine.

As I will show, the case of Victoria Terrell helped to define the attributes that determined which overseas doctors could become full members of British medicine. In 1965 Terrell violated the temporality condition of her registration by becoming a naturalized citizen as a consequence of marrying a British national.[1] Even though this provision of the 1948 Medical Act was designed to discourage the settlement of overseas doctors, supporters of Terrell portrayed her as a victim of an obsolete registration system that penalized service to the public and rewarded unearned entitlement. Terrell's case was not simply about repealing the temporality clause; it was equally about which overseas doctors could assimilate and embody British medicine. Rather than subverting the white and largely male social identity of British medicine, Terrell's European origins, English-language competency, gender, and marriage were highly compatible with it as well as with the sexual division of labor in the profession. Indeed, women accounted for 15 percent of the profession and tended to be concentrated in general practice and in pediatrics, among other low prestige specialties.[2] At the same time, this set of attributes contrasted with a well-worn set of stereotypes about south Asian male doctors that emphasized their alterity. Their transient relationship to Britain—once a source of reassurance about their intentions—had become a liability and was seen now as evidence of a lack of commitment to British medicine. The British public questioned the English-language skills of overseas-trained doctors, their capacity to assimilate, and their ability to safely practice medicine. Even as British medicine became more politicized, the GMC defended its administration of the register and the competency of overseas-trained doctors. But this position proved to be a short-lived one. Fee revenue from the registration of overseas doctors became unreliable as criticism steadily mounted and their admission to the register began to decline. The council's position began to diverge from its public actions when it shifted financial responsibility for funding the GMC from overseas doctors to domestic medical graduates.

The Domestic Globalization of British Medicine, 1955–66

As Britain entered the postwar period, returning the domestic output of medical graduates to replacement levels increasingly became a priority. This was not entirely a surprise. Structurally, the legal relationship between medical qualifications awarded in the United Kingdom and admission to the British register meant that the capacity of university and nonuniversity licensing bodies limited the growth of the profession. It is mainly for this reason that medical bodies took steps to increase the production of doctors during the national emergences of total war. Barely cracked before World War I, they opened their portals to women in significant numbers to help manage the personnel demands of the military and the needs of the civilian population. With the return to peacetime in 1919, they narrowed their portals to women while allowing the intake and output to return to approximate parity during the inter-war period. During World War II, medical schools not only abbreviated the length of instruction but also expanded their intake of medical students to produce more doctors. As in the inter-war period, in the postwar period also constraint, rather than expansion, animated the domestic intake of medical students and output of medical graduates to a significant degree.

This was the essence of the recommendation of the Commission to Consider the Future Numbers of Medical Practitioners and the Appropriate Intake of Medical Students in 1957. Chaired by Sir Henry Willink, the commission was charged with forecasting the long-term medical personnel needs of the United Kingdom. The commission narrowed its forecasting time horizon to the decade from 1961 to 1971.[3] This horizon grounded future supply trends in relation to the absorption of doctors currently in medical school or otherwise unavailable before 1961. Conceding their limited capacity to forecast beyond a decade due to the "imponderables" of population growth and the nature of demand for health care, a ten-year period seemed to provide a far more realistic time horizon.[4] Meanwhile, the committee projected a slight surplus of doctors based on the difference between projected departures, forecasted expansion and planned requirements of the armed services and the output of medical schools in Britain and Northern Ireland.[5] This surplus, together with the availability of short-term and National Service doctors in the existing services, added 1,060 for civilian practice. The committee was fairly confident that this surplus would enable Britain to fill existing deficiencies (780) in civilian practices.[6]

Looking beyond the current supply and demand, the committee took a far different view of the next decade (see table 5.1). The commission recommended a 10 percent reduction in the medical school intake beginning in 1961.[7] Driving their recommendation was diminishing opportunity or, at least, relatively stable domestic staffing needs. The committee projected 4 percent growth in the general population. The needs of the military shrunk in response to the postwar geopolitical landscape, reacting to decolonization in the empire and the security provided by the US-led North American Treaty Alliance. Only an annual intake of fifty doctors to the armed services was deemed necessary to replace projected retirements and death among permanent officers. At the same time, the committee was confident about the declining loss of domestic medical graduates due to out-migration. By 1971 the annual departures, the panel forecasted, would decline from 160 in 1955 to fifty.

Regarding in-migration from overseas countries, the committee also painted a reassuring picture of stability: high demand for study in Britain but relatively low demand for settling permanently. After initially absorbing foreign doctors on the temporary register to the full register following the war, the report noted that "since about 1950 the number of foreign trained

Table 5.1. Total average annual medical labor requirements, 1955–71

Replacement of wastage by	Mid-1955–mid-1960	Mid-1960–mid-1965	Mid-1965–mid-1970	Mid-1970–mid-1971
Death and retirement	1150	1180	1230	1260
Expansion	465	440	280	280
Armed Forces	55	55	55	55
"Export"	160	110	70	50
Total	1830	1785	1635	1645

Source: Report of Committee to Consider the Future Numbers of Medical Practitioners and the Appropriate Intake of Medical Students (London: Her Majesty's Stationery Office, 1957), 32.

doctors admitted to the Foreign List and taking up residence here has been insignificant and it is probable that most of that small number come here only for post-graduate study and experience and will in due course return to their own countries." This pattern persisted for the majority of doctors trained in the Commonwealth. Settling in Britain was not a high priority. The "number of doctors from the Commonwealth at present settling here each year is about 75."[8]

Given these estimates, the committee concluded a gross intake of 1,760 of domestic medical graduates annually would yield a net output of 1,955 when combined with the in-migration of overseas-trained doctors.[9] Although shortly after the publication of the committee report, the recommendation was roundly criticized for underestimating staffing demand, the intake trend indicates that medical schools conformed to the recommendation until 1965.[10] The overall intake of medical students would not recover to the 1958 peak until 1971. Between 1958 and 1961 alone, the intake plunged 21 percent. Thereafter, the year over year increase stayed within a 1 percent to 2 percent range. The 9 percent increase in 1965 was the effect of a government expansion plan.[11] It called for restoring the 10 percent reduction and an additional increase of 150 students by 1966. In support of this increase, plans for the construction of a medical school at Nottingham University were brought forward. But the impact of the new medical school would not bear fruit until it opened in 1969 and the graduation of its first cohort in 1974. Given the time lag between intake and graduation, the aggregate output of medical graduates slowly changed (see table 5.2).

Registration trends between 1955 and 1966 reflected the lag effect of the slow recovery of the intake of medical students and the growth in overseas sources of admissions to the register.[12] The supply of British and Irish admissions—originating from England, Scotland, and Ireland—was stable, averaging

Table 5.2. Medical students beginning preclinical courses at medical schools in Great Britain, 1961–72

British-based students	England	Great Britain	Other students	England	Great Britain
1961	1371	1788		143	232
1962	1406	1896		130	207
1963	1550	2035		112	157
1964	1627	2166		83	115
1965	1693	2257		103	150
1966	1728	2312		110	166
1967	1777	2391		67	111
1968	1823	2442		71	118
1969	1931	2547		102	146
1970	1919	2582		83	113
1971	2105	2770		79	108
1972	2114	2929		75	103

Source: Medical Manpower Table, MH 149/1828.

2,212 during the period. The total annual number oscillated between 2,305 in 1955 and 2,163 in 1966. The trend for provisional registration was similarly stable.[13] Full admissions of British and Irish graduates totaled 23,598 and averaged 1,966 annually. When overseas graduates were added to this category of the registration, the total increased to 40,500 and the annual average to 3,375. The total number of overseas graduates (4,406) was lower than domestic graduates because the pool of candidates who sought full registration was generally drawn from a limited number of reciprocating countries. Still, their numbers impressively increased 89 percent between 1955 and 1966 while accounting for 15 percent of all admissions (see table 5.3).

Of the two routes to the register, requalification yielded the smallest numbers. Between 1957 and 1966, 568 requalified for an average of 56 annually. These doctors originated from countries throughout the world. Regionally, South Asia accounted for the largest proportion (29.9 percent), followed closely by Europe (29 percent) and the Middle East (25 percent) (see table 5.4). Overseas doctors with recognized medical qualifications from reciprocating countries registered in far greater numbers than those who requalified.

Table 5.3. Postwar registration statistics: provincial and full registration for England, Scotland, Ireland, and Commonwealth countries, 1955–66

Commonwealth and foreign	1955	1956	1957	1958	1959	1960	1961	1962	1963	1964	1965	1966
Provisional	87	107	109	145	308	464	473	419	277	523	678	816
Temporary	775	1086	1294	1319	1477	1701	1965	2094	2595	2922	3236	3551
English												
Full	1562	1560	1571	1480	1418	1431	1446	1519	1512	1441	1412	1510
Provisional	1526	1594	1454	1541	1446	1465	1453	1420	1432	1425	1397	1483
Scottish												
Full	395	442	487	433	472	436	429	426	353	394	394	371
Provisional	464	486	429	450	447	457	432	371	372	382	392	453
Irish												
Full	348	348	336	366	325	282	288	244	295	251	295	282
Provisional	82	87	70	68	54	66	58	58	61	76	69	78

Source: Registration Statistics, section 2 of appendix 1 from General Medical Council, Memorandum on the Registration of Commonwealth and Foreign Doctors, October 1967, MH 153/548.

Table 5.4. Postwar registration statistics: requalification, 1957–66

	1957	1958	1959	1960	1961	1962	1963	1964	1965	1966	Total
Europe	12	13	31	18	14	14	12	21	15	16	166
Middle East											
Egypt Sudan	5	4	5	14	9	22	18	17	26	24	144
Iraq											
Other	1	—	1	2	—	—	3	5	1	4	16
Africa	2	1	1	1	—	1	—	—	—	—	6
South Asia											
India											
Pakistan	9	7	16	23	33	30	22	10	15	5	170
Burma											
Far East	2	5	3	4	8	8	8	9	4	7	58
United States	1	2	—	—	—	1	—	1	1	1	7
South America	—	—	—	—	1	—	—	—	—	—	1
Totals	32	32	57	61	65	76	63	63	62	57	568

Source: Requalification table A in appendix 5, General Medical Council, Memorandum on the Registration of Commonwealth and Foreign Doctors, October 1967, MH 153/548.

Table 5.5. Postwar admissions to the British Medial Register from Commonwealth countries: Full registration

Country	1955	1956	1957	1958	1959	1960	1961	1962	1963	1964	1965	1966	Total
Australia	238	189	192	175	189	181	225	176	198	205	274	239	2481
Burma	5	5	14	18	36	27	32	33	36	22	16	21	265
Canada	29	46	54	55	71	60	64	49	62	62	55	54	661
Ceylon	19	23	44	65	60	47	98	62	86	101	115	111	831
East Africa	—	—	—	7	13	8	4	8	9	11	17	12	89
Hong Kong	12	17	11	17	34	27	32	32	30	18	36	41	307
India	170	287	344	399	429	591	678	482	388	389	623	702	5482
Malaysia	6	9	10	12	20	13	26	19	19	24	43	26	227
Malta	1	5	12	5	8	13	10	2	10	9	2	14	91
New Zealand	44	59	35	65	53	46	62	54	53	54	59	39	623
Pakistan	20	19	31	64	61	109	86	79	89	160	203	288	1209
South Africa	119	103	84	98	78	202	449	303	69	52	66	57	1680
Totals	663	762	831	980	1052	1324	1766	1299	1049	1107	1509	1604	13946

Source: Requalification table A in appendix 5, General Medical Council, Memorandum on the Registration of Commonwealth and Foreign Doctors, October 1967, MH 153/548.

Some 13,946 doctors from twelve Commonwealth countries or territories were admitted. After 1955 the supply of doctors from India exceeded those from "Old" Commonwealth countries Australia, Canada, New Zealand, and South Africa, among others, and accounted for at least one-third or more of doctors in this category. Pakistan edged ahead of Canada in 1960, New Zealand in 1961, and South Africa in 1963. South Asian countries together—India, Pakistan, and Burma—accounted for 49 percent of all admissions to the register (see table 5.5).

The growth trend for admissions to the register through temporary registration was even more robust.[14] The total number of temporary registrants (24,015) approximated the total number for both domestic provisional (23,598) and full registration (26,554). The category of temporary registration alone accounted for 32 percent of all admissions to the register. The proportion of temporary registration in relation to all categories of registration grew from 14 percent in 1955 to 41 percent in 1966. The rate of increase at the start and end of the period was much greater as well. Annual admissions rose from 775 in 1955 to 3,551 in 1966, or 70 percent. Provisional registration grew far more modestly at 21 percent. The rate for fully registered doctors actually declined.

The category of temporary registration exhibited regional variation between Europe and the Commonwealth and among Commonwealth countries (see table 5.6). The total number of temporary registration certificates awarded was 2,276 and 2,450 respectively in 1965 and 1966. In 1965 Europe accounted for 28 percent, Africa 22 percent, Asia 39 percent, and northern and southern Africa 9 percent. In the following year, there was slight change: Europe accounted for 33 percent, Africa 18 percent, Asia 39 percent, and North and South America 8 percent. Within regions, several individual countries stood out as posting the largest number of certificates: Greece and Spain in Europe, Egypt in Africa, India and Pakistan in Asia, and the United States and Brazil in North and South America. This regional pattern was consistent for those who obtained temporary registration for the first time (see table 5.7). In 1965 and 1966, Europe accounted for 34 percent and 34 percent, Africa 16 percent and 14 percent, Asia 31 percent and 35 percent, and North and South America 18 percent and 17 percent. The countries with the largest number of registered doctors also remained consistent: Greece and Poland in Europe; Egypt in Africa; India, Iraq, and Pakistan in Asia; and the United States and Brazil in North and South America.

These trends were indicative of the global profile of postwar British medicine.[15] In the centennial year of the founding of the GMC, council president Sir David Campbell highlighted the ways in which British medicine was a model for the world. Its standards of regulating the profession served, he stated, as "a model or indeed a mother of all the medical councils in the Commonwealth. The statutes establishing them had been based on and have

Table 5.6. Postwar admissions to the British Medical Register: temporary registration, 1965–66

Country	1965	1966
Europe		
Austria	1	6
Belgium	4	14
Bulgaria	4	5
Czechoslovakia	13	33
Denmark	4	3
Finland	3	3
France	12	21
East Germany	0	5
West Germany	6	18
Greece	266	343
Hungary	10	11
Iceland	15	5
Italy	36	54
Netherlands	4	3
Norway	4	4
Poland	39	63
Portugal	22	22
Romania	1	9
Spain	153	140
Sweden	0	2
Switzerland	29	24
USSR	2	9
Yugoslavia	23	22
Total	651	814
[%] Total Qualified	29%	33%

(continued)

Table 5.6.—*(continued)*

Country	1965	1966
North and South America		
Argentina	17	15
Bolivia	2	1
Brazil	16	25
Canada	41	35
Chile	4	7
Colombia	8	4
Dominican Republic	42	
Ecuador	2	3
El Salvador	1	9
Guatemala	1	1
Haiti	1	0
Mexico	12	12
Nicaragua	0	0
Panama	1	2
Peru	4	9
Uruguay	1	0
USA	90	75
Venezuela	5	4
Total	210	204
[%] Total Qualified	9%	8%
Asia		
Afghanistan	5	5
Burma	7	2
China	2	0
India	266	270

(continued)

Table 5.6.—*(concluded)*

Country	1965	1966
Iran	117	127
Iraq	146	179
Israel	8	8
Japan	7	7
South Korea	2	1
Lebanon	14	31
Pakistan	195	160
Philippines	14	22
Syria	47	64
Thailand	16	17
Turkey	63	72
Total	909	968
[%] Total Qualified	40%	40%
Africa		
Nigeria	0	1
Sudan	24	28
Egypt	482	435
Total	506	464
[%] Total Qualified	22%	19%

Source: Admission to the British Medical Register section 3a of appendix 1 Certifications of Registration, General Medical Council, Memorandum on the Registration of Commonwealth and Foreign Doctors, October 1967, MH 153/548.

often copied verbatim the words of the British Medical Acts."[16] The education and ethical norms wove the profession of medicine closely together. The visitations and advice of the council ensured common standards and spurred the expansion of needed medical training. Sir David noted that granting temporary recognition to new schools was a risk that had yielded benefits: "It led in every case to a striking improvement in the provision of facilities for education and in the standard of attainment."[17] Lord Cohen

Table 5.7. Postwar admissions to the British Medical Register: first-time temporary registration, 1965–66

Europe	1965	1966
Austria	1	2
Belgium	1	8
Bulgaria	2	2
Czechoslovakia	13	15
Denmark	3	3
Finland	3	1
France	4	8
East Germany	1	0
West Germany	5	7
Greece	62	89
Hungary	4	2
Iceland	2	2
Italy	15	14
Netherlands	3	1
Norway	3	2
Poland	24	29
Portugal	7	8
Romania	0	3
Spain	40	30
Sweden	0	2
Switzerland	12	9
USSR	0	2
Yugoslavia	10	6
Total	215	245
[%] Total Qualified	35%	35%

(continued)

Table 5.7.—*(continued)*

North and South America	1965	1966
Argentina	5	6
Bolivia	1	0
Brazil	9	12
Canada	21	23
Chile	9	9
Colombia	2	1
Dominican Republic	20	
Ecuador	0	1
El Salvador	1	2
Mexico	7	4
Nicaragua	0	0
Panama	1	1
Peru	2	7
Uruguay	1	0
USA	54	45
Venezuela	3	3
Total	112	108
[%] Total Qualified	18%	13%
Asia		
Afghanistan	3	2
Burma	0	2
China	0	1
India	33	67
Iran	28	28
Iraq	35	53
Israel	6	7

(continued)

Table 5.7.—*(concluded)*

Asia	1965	1966
Japan	4	4
South Korea	0	1
Lebanon	5	7
Pakistan	39	30
Philippines	6	7
Syria	8	18
Thailand	11	6
Turkey	16	18
Total	194	251
[%] Total Qualified	31%	36%
Africa		
Nigeria	0	1
Sudan	8	9
Egypt	93	94
Total	101	103
[%] Total Qualified	16%	15%

Source: Section 3b of appendix 1 Certifications of Registration, General Medical Council, Memorandum on the Registration of Commonwealth and Foreign Doctors, October 1967, MH 153/548.

of Birkenhead, Sir David's successor and the first Jew to be council president, added that "reciprocity in registration and temporary registration was one of the most abiding links of friendship with the Commonwealth."[18] If anything, the increasing numbers of overseas and foreign doctors on the temporary register was a source of pride. Cohen said as much in his 1965 presidential address. "The figures left no doubt as to the weighty contribution of this country to the postgraduate training of overseas doctors, not from the British Commonwealth only, but also from many foreign countries in all parts of the globe."[19]

The benefits of overseas migration translated into a significant source of revenue for the GMC as well (see table 5.8). By the early 1960s, growth

Table 5.8. Postwar sources of revenue: Commonwealth and foreign registration fees and other, 1965–68

Publication sales	1965	1966	1967	1968
Copy of Medical Register	5268	6343	8614	6692
List of names and sundry publications	1996	1907	1853	1832
Total publications	7265	8250	10468	8524
British Pharmacopeia				
Charge for office services	1000	1000	1000	1000
Fees (Commonwealth and foreign) for full, provisional, and temporary registration				
Full at £21	22701	21672	24990	30723
Full after provisional at £12	5136	6864	7608	9072
Provisional at £9	6102	7344	7317	7965
Temporary at £3 10s.	4000	4553	5922	8796
Temporary at £10	20930	22500	26610	33624
Certificates of good standing at £2	1100	1158	1264	1910
Additional qualifications at £1	691	258	176	141
Public health diplomas at £2	52	12	12	4
Change in name at £1	35	48	41	48
Restorations at £2	16	276	160	74
Certified copies of entry at £1	36	31	40	61
Search sees at £1	—	—	—	85
Total fees	60794	64725	74246	92540
Dividends and interest	1300	1003	1355	1137
Contributed by branch councils (rounded)				
English Branch Council	11369	12455	11114	29488
Scottish Branch Council	3363	3504	3351	8651
Irish Branch Council	1683	1761	1693	4263
Total branch contributions	16377	17719	16159	42403
Total income and contributions	86735	92697	103228	145604

Source: Figures rounded to the nearest pound. Adapted from Income and Expenditure Account Statement from Annual Accounts Report, 1965–68, *Minutes of the General Medical Council of Education and Registration* (London: General Medical Council, 1965–69).

complicated the capacity of the GMC to carry out its statutory responsibilities. This meant processing more doctors for registration, monitoring medical education—especially the operation of the mandated preregistration year posts—and adjudicating disciplinary cases. Operating costs covered a range of categories. These included fees and expenses for members, printing, office expenses, correction of the register, legal expenses, and visitation and inspection of examinations and medical schools in the United Kingdom and overseas. Between 1948 and 1964, these and other costs increased fourfold, from 22,763 pounds in 1948 to 46,695 pounds in 1956 and finally to 95,133 pounds in 1964.[20] This increase was linked to trends in the postwar economy. Inflation reduced the value of the pound and translated into higher labor costs, such as wages and salaries, national insurance contributions, and office rents and rates. Against these costs, the sources of revenue were relatively limited.[21] The largest sources included the sale of publications and the *British Pharmacopaeia*, fees from overseas doctors' registration and fees associated with the registration of United Kingdom medical graduates. Of these sources, registration fees were by far the single largest source of revenue.

Over the 1965–1968 period, the GMC generated 428,264 pounds from all sources. Of these three sources, revenue from publications (the medical register and other publications) rose modestly at best, from 7,265 pounds in 1965, peaking at 10,468 pounds in 1967, then back down to 8,524 pounds in 1968. The *British Pharmacopaeia* yielded a reliable 1,000 per year for office charges. Together these sources totaled 47,416 pounds over the four-year period or 5 percent of the total revenue. The fee income category produced 292,305 pounds in revenue, or 70 percent during the same period. The contributions from the branch council accounted for 109,308 pounds, or 12 percent of total income.

While registration fees were important overall, there were significance differences between those related to domestic and overseas medical graduates. The fees for domestic graduates were one time only—at the time of admission to the register. Until 1950 the initial fee of five pounds had remained in place since 1858. To the extent that these fees were one time, they comprised a constant source of revenue that was related to the annual number of medical graduates. With authorization from the Privy Council, the council in 1950 increased the initial registration fee to six pounds, six shillings, while provisional registration was set at five pounds, five shillings, or eleven pounds for full registration after the completion of the preregistration period.[22]

Fees derived from applicants for temporary registration proved to be a far more elastic source of revenue. The nature of these fees differed from those associated with provisional and initial registration in two important ways. Temporary registration was of limited duration and had to be renewed at the end of the scheduled expiration of the certificate in order to be employed in an approved hospital or institution. The council was in a position to collect fees more than once from the same person. Second, the total amount of these fees was not fixed to the number of medical graduates but subject to the supply of overseas doctors seeking to work or train in Britain. Third, the GMC collected additional fees from overseas and foreign trained doctors, unlike graduates of United Kingdom institutions. These included certificates of good standing, public health diplomas, changes of name, restorations, and certified copies of entry. Between 1964 and 1969, the fee revenue for overseas medical graduates was invariably at least two times that of their United Kingdom counterparts.[23]

While these fees made up for shortcomings in other revenue sources, they were not able to place the GMC on a stable footing. Given the reliance on fee revenue from overseas doctors, any sharp changes in the supply and demand for overseas doctors increased the risk of operating on a deficit. The operation of the 1962 Commonwealth Immigration Act had this effect. The act, which Parliament passed in response to growing opposition to the pace and scale of immigration from "new" Commonwealth countries, mandated that all nonnationals possess a voucher as a condition to enter the country to work. Reflecting the duality of immigration policy—domestic needs and international relevance—the act provided exemptions for critical areas, including medicine, while privileging residents from the "old" Commonwealth. The effect of the act on the flow of doctors mirrored general immigration. Among donor countries such as India and Pakistan, the year before passage witnessed a significant increase in the number of doctors obtaining full registration, followed by a two-year drop in admits after implementation before recovering in 1964 (see table 5.5).[24] Contextualizing the trends of overseas doctors was the migration of domestic medical graduates outside of the United Kingdom. For critics of the system of registration, not to mention the NHS, their movement highlighted the distorted incentives of the globalization of British medicine.

Tensions at the Heart of British Medicine: The Migration of Overseas Doctors to Britain and the Emigration of British Doctors

The trend in the registration of overseas doctors paralleled the mobility of domestic medical graduates. After the nineteenth century, only a self-selected group of doctors had migrated to other countries or the empire. Many of those who left Britain did so primarily because of limited prospects in the domestic market and opportunities in fast-growing settler colonies. Still others sought the relative security of a salaried appointment in the public services such as the Army Medical Service, Indian Medical Services, or the Colonial Medical Services, among others.[25] By the interwar period, a combination of the growing indigenous production of practitioners in destination countries in the Commonwealth and a more favorable doctor-to-population ratio in Britain checked the flow of migration.[26] After the war, the pattern changed in important ways. Estimates for the annual average outflow of British medical graduates between 1955 and 1960 ranged from 483 to 650—the equivalent of nearly one-third of all medical school graduates.[27] Their destinations included reciprocating Commonwealth countries with sizable white populations such as Australia, South Africa, and New Zealand. North America, especially the United States and Canada, became a major destination for British doctors.

The meaning of occupational migration became a focal point of discussion in the British medical press by the late 1950s. Rather than acknowledging mobility as a long-standing strategy of domestic medical graduates, articles instead portrayed this migration in the context of the skepticism of organized medicine toward postwar socialized medicine. For critics of the NHS, migration afforded evidence of the inadequacy of career prospects in private practice or hospital service for British-educated doctors. The regulation of private practice (to ensure an even distribution of doctors) by local medical boards narrowed options, as did the requirement that new doctors serve as assistants to retiring doctors as a condition of entering a new practice. In addition, rules governing patient lists, together with government-regulated fees for services, added to a sense of overwork and financial insecurity for private practices. Hospital service was hardly better. Staffing in the hospital was divided between preregistered and registered posts, which were aligned to general and specialized areas of practice. All doctors had to complete a yearlong house officer position—six months in general medicine and six months in general surgery or midwifery. Thereafter, registered house officer posts as well as those for junior and senior registrars in specialties reflected availability; higher qualification; and, above all, the confidence of the supervising consultant. The chronically low number of consultant positions meant protracted periods of service in house and registrar posts with little chance of promotion to the apex of the career hierarchy.[28]

The disconnection between the training needs of practitioners and the labor requirements of hospitals stunted career development. High demand for hospital services impaired the growth of formal postgraduate training and research-intensive careers, especially in nonteaching hospitals. To be sure, the Nuffield Regional Provincial Hospitals Trust subsidized training in nonteaching hospitals, especially in northern England and Scotland, through cooperation with regional hospital groups, general practitioners, and junior medical staff. Sponsored lectures, seminars, and informal clinical meetings did not alter the fact that established urban-based teaching hospitals, which were associated with universities, remained the main gateways for university- and hospital-based research and specialist careers.[29]

It was in this context that the movement of domestic and overseas medical graduates became politically visible. The "Report of the Joint Working Group on the Structure of Medical Staffing in the Hospital Service" dissected the structural defects of the service.[30] Chaired by Sir Robert Platt, the Group reached a number of findings that confirmed the perception of a national service in crisis. British medical graduates on average spent three years in the junior grades, including their intern year: 36 percent remained in the service for less than two years, 29 percent for less than three and 35 percent for three years or more. Overseas doctors filled this shortage of British-born doctors. "Of the 9,543 employed 3,236, or almost 36 percent, qualified outside Great Britain and a large number (3,628) were born outside Great Britain,"[31] the Report said. Sir Robert emphasized the importance of addressing the staffing needs of the service from indigenous sources as the relationship between Britain and donor countries was liable to change: "While we hope that many young doctors from overseas will continue to come to this country for postgraduate training, we must not ignore the probability of some decline in that number as arrangements for postgraduate training are developed in their own countries."[32]

Conversely, the exit of both experienced and recently qualified doctors from the national service was raised in Parliament. In the House of Commons, Commander J. S. Kerans queried the Conservative health minister Enoch Powell about the number of general practitioners who stopped participating in the NHS. Powell reported that 4,350 doctors withdrew from NHS general practice contracts—without discussing the reasons for the separations. Kerans not only volunteered that they were due to the "overladen capacity of work that they had to do and the frustration of administration" but also insinuated that the non-British doctors were replacing them. He asked Powell if it would be possible to "get more doctors from the Commonwealth and elsewhere to supplement the present deficiencies in the Health Service." Evading Kerans's question, Powell noted that "the number of general practitioners on the Health Service lists is increasing."[33]

The publication of "Medical Emigration from Britain, 1930–1961," by John Seale, a health economist, proved to be embarrassing to the government. Seale rendered the general dissatisfaction with career prospects quantitatively.[34] A study of the names of British graduates on medical registers in New Zealand, Australia, South Africa, Southern and Northern Rhodesia, and the United States produced a startling observation: there had been a "mass migration of British doctors in the last fifteen years away from their native land on a scale hitherto unknown." Placing the three-decade average in context, Seale reported that "the average of over 600 registering annually in these countries alone is equivalent to a third of the annual output of the medical schools of Great Britain and Ireland." The cause of this pattern was clear enough: "Practice in the National Medical Service is relatively unattractive to young doctors economically, professionally, and idealistically." The short- and long-term consequences of migration jeopardized the very idea of a national service. Seale pointed out that relying on overseas doctors was no solution since "most come to Britain to enhance their professional standing and then return to their own country—few intend to remain in Britain permanently." Nor did the indigenous supply of medical graduates bode well for the future. The supply of medical students declined from 14,201 in 1950 to 12,314 in 1959, which was only 431 above the number in 1938." As if to underscore the declining appeal of medicine as a career, Seale added that "there are 625 fewer male medical students in 1959 than in 1938."[35]

Seale's reference to male doctors simultaneously underscored the persistence of gender privilege within British medicine and exposed the under use of women doctors. A de facto quota limited the enrollment of women in medical schools to a national average of 25 percent after 1945. By 1964 women medical graduates accounted for a quarter of all domestic medical graduates admitted to the register and a fifth of the total profession.[36] Yet their participation in the profession lagged in proportion to their availability. The Federation of Medical Women and others pointed out hurdles and barriers that limited the participation of women doctors. These included sexism in the selection of training positions and career structures that did not accommodate part-time work or reentry for married women doctors with families. Advocates of gender equity emphasized the utilization of women doctors as part of the solution to the staffing needs of the NHS. "Much has been said of the loss of doctors by emigration," A. H. T. Robb-Smith volunteered, "but little cognizance has been taken of the increasing wastage of women doctors." He added "at a conservative estimate, there are at present time five thousand medical women, mostly between the ages of thirty and forty-five, who are not in practice, and those who qualified in the past twenty years are fortunate if they spend eight years in their profession—not a very good return for a five-year training which costs the taxpayer some ten thousand pounds."[37]

The government's defensive response to Searle's analysis also reinforced the racial and gender composition of the NHS, and by extension British medicine, as normatively white and male. Addressing the Annual Conference of Representatives of Local Medical Committees, Powell cast doubt on the scale of emigration:[38] "Data from a dozen medical schools in London and the provinces show that of British doctors who graduated from them during the 1950s the proportion who are resident abroad is between 6 and 7%."[39] Turning the meaning of the mobility of British doctors on its head, Powell regarded travel as a quintessential sign of a modern society and profession, not a means to hollow out the character of the profession.[40]

In questioning Seale's analysis, Powell opened himself to further queries from the House. Kenneth Robinson (St. Pancras, North) called for more reliable statistics on the supply and choices of domestic medical graduates.[41] Powell saw no need, asserting that the overall increase in domestically trained hospital medical staff exceeded the absolute increase of overseas doctors in the service as well as their total numbers overall: "These figures completely refuted the notion that work in the Health Service was not attractive to graduates of British medical schools; their numbers were increasing in every branch."[42] Letters and editorials published in the medical press contradicted Powell's description. Emigration remained an option, according to M. H. Pappworth, because of the dearth of posts at teaching hospitals leading to a hospital consultancy.[43]

A lead article in the *British Medical Journal* declared, "This country is losing more doctors than it can spare. It is at the same time, and partly because of this, having to staff N.H.S. hospitals with doctors from abroad whose training has been different from those educated in British medical schools, and whose work in any case is inadequately supervised."[44] Britain was experiencing a drain of its best graduates. Referring to a recent report by Abel-Smith and Gale that documented occupational emigration, it noted that the authors of the report "found that about two-thirds of British-born doctors engaged in this kind of academic work in the U.S.A. had been trained in London and Oxford and Cambridge." The article concluded that the drain was a national crisis. "All concerned with the welfare of Medicine should take heed of these and other warnings. It is no good having a free Health Service unless it is a good service. If conditions continue to be such as to cause emigration on the present scale, the standards of medical practice are bound gradually to deteriorate."[45] The public and now explicit link between a presumptive good service and domestic medical graduates staffing it implied that the presence of overseas doctors in British hospitals did not augur well for the NHS or, by extension, the public. This amounted to a significant shift in the relationship of overseas doctors to British medicine. Encouraged to train in the United Kingdom, they had come in significant numbers, far exceeding the supply of domestic medical graduates added to the register. Their registration fees subsidized the operations of the GMC while their labor enabled the state to deliver medical care to the British public. Against the emerging discourse on national depletion in the early 1960s, however, they were judged by their capacity to fit into a far more narrow definition of British medicine. The medium that had globalized postwar British medicine—the medical register—became a lightning rod for scrutiny and criticism.

Recasting the Boundaries of British Medicine: The Victoria Terrell Case

More so than any single event, the Victoria Terrell case provided an occasion for openly discussing recasting the boundaries of British medicine.

At issue was the capacity of overseas doctors not only to practice medicine, but also to assimilate within society. Originally qualified in Warsaw in 1961, Dr. Victoria Jasiewicz specialized in pediatrics after completing her internship and obtaining her medical diploma.[46] In February 1963, she traveled to Britain and applied to the GMC for temporary registration. Until 1966 Jasiewicz's experience was unremarkable. She received certificates in April and June 1964 and May 1965. The council included in her 1965 certificate an "early warning letter." The purpose of this communication underscored the temporality of registration, which the council limited to a maximum of five years.

> You will understand therefore that, if you later wish to obtain a further period of registration, the Council will require you to submit, together with or preferably in advance of your application, a detailed statement in writing of the purpose for which you are proposing to continue to reside in the United Kingdom. In particular, you should then state whether you are seeking to obtain any postgraduate qualifications, and, if so, what progress you have made, up to the date of your letter, and when you expect to take the relevant examination. You should also state the approximate data (year and month) by which you are proposing to leave the United Kingdom.[47]

Between this communication and November 1966, Jasiewicz married Christopher Terrell and changed her name. In November her husband wrote on her behalf seeking information about full registration. In reply the council provided information about the procedure to obtain a primary qualification from one of the three nonuniversity licensing bodies. By securing such a qualification in the United Kingdom, Terrell would be eligible for provisional registration and full registration after completing the year-long preregistration appointment—unless exempted.[48] The opportunity costs associated with requalification in the United Kingdom—interruption of professional activity and gainful employment—was clearly designed to discourage overseas doctors on the temporary register from pursuing full registration.

Within months, Terrell's registration status opened a wider discussion about the defects in the system of temporary registration. *The Lancet*'s "Marriage and the G.M.C." informed readers that Terrell "has a Polish degree and her temporary registration was withdrawn when she became British by marriage."[49] Her predicament was not an isolated one but rather "illustrated the distinction which is made between graduates of Commonwealth and those from other countries." While acknowledging that "good historical reasons for reciprocity" existed, the article went on to describe how postwar conditions made reciprocity an artifact of the past. "The upsurge of new medical schools in Asia, however, has been such that the G.M.C. now has to exercise a continuous process of acceptance or rejection—in which rejection has so far predominated." Rather than assuring the maintenance of a British standard of medical education and training, reciprocity in the era of decolonization lowered standards. Unlike doctors from Asia whose applications for registration were rejected by the council, Terrell's qualifications and experience were presumed to be satisfactory because she worked in a clinical setting under the direct supervision of the senior British medical staff. "Surely it is ludicrous that when a doctor declares an intention to remain in Great Britain the reward is a decree of unfitness to practice here."[50]

A follow-up article set temporary registration against reciprocity to underscore the "justice" for registration reform. Britain benefited a great deal from overseas doctors. Their labor contributed to the delivery of health care to the British public. But it remained unclear whether they returned home with the desired experience or qualifications that motivated them to travel to the United Kingdom. Tacitly acknowledging their exploitation, the article added, "The only way this country can justify benefiting by all of this professional help, which might otherwise be given to people in greater need, is to ensure that these doctors are satisfactorily trained." By contrast, this sense of obligation was not extended to doctors who were eligible to be registered under reciprocity arrangements. These doctors came to Britain not out of altruism or educational need but out of self-serving careerism. They exploited an obsolete system of regulating the movement of doctors. When "strictly supervised," there were advantages to reciprocity, such as the "maintenance of high standards of medical education and the free exchange of medical graduates." But in the wake of the rapid growth of medical schools, the demand for doctors, and the comparative ease of travel facilitating the movement of doctors to Britain, the provisions of reciprocity tied the hands of the council to "strictly" assess them for their medical fitness. This created a double standard for overseas doctors. The temporarily registered were subject to narrowly defined restrictions, while those who were entitled to practice medicine were treated as if they were domestic medical graduates when they were trained beyond the territorial reach of Great Britain. The article concluded that "justice must be simultaneously and plainly seen to be achieved on behalf of doctors from non-reciprocal countries who wish to make a career in Britain; and, as things stand at the moment, that vision is occasionally blurred."[51]

In its overview of temporary registration, *The Lancet* focused on the procedure of overseas registration itself and, in so doing, questioned the council's capacity to assess the fitness of applicants.[52] Although authorized to screen medical diplomas and degrees of applicants, the task was next to impossible. Keeping up with the growth in number of medical schools worldwide—estimated to be six hundred in 1960—was exacerbated by the lack of reliable information about them. "The Council's task in this respect is not made easier by the variation of standards within the country and at different times,"[53] *The Lancet* article remarked. For this reason, it refused to accept some qualifications granted in Indonesia and China. Beyond this blanket refusal, the council designated qualifications either "acceptable" or "unacceptable." While these designations implied an unproblematic determination of credentials and medical fitness, the precise nature of their meaning was left to the discretion of the council. In other words, the evaluative process was more art than science. Rather than minimizing this impression, the council's "safeguards" reinforced it. Applicants whose qualifications were deemed acceptable or unacceptable either received certificates limited to "posts in hospitals for pre-registration purposes" or were asked to provide "evidence of postgraduate training" if the requested post appeared beyond their training. The role of English-language competency underscored the subjective nature, if not loose oversight, of the registration process. The council reserved the right to deny registration in cases when it "doubted whether an applicant's English is sufficient for the job he is proposing to do." But this was no guarantee. "A substantial proportion of doctors do present themselves at the London office of the G.M.C. at some point during their stay; but the G.M.C. need not necessarily be in verbal touch with an applicant, and written applications are not always a reliable guide." Nor were standards of English-language competence consistent: "Moreover, an understaffed hospital in the North of England is not likely to complain about a houseman's English unless this is quite intolerable."[54]

The medical press coverage generated letters to the editor that reinforced the call for reform precisely by drawing attention to the disparities or other effects associated with reciprocity. For G. D. Pirrie, the prescribed number of countries narrowed Britain's access to accomplished doctors while producing manifest anomalies. "Are the graduates of Oxford and Otago always so much better than those doctors from Tokyo and Toronto. Delhi and Dublin than Berlin and Basle? Are Abana and Pharpar always to be preferred?"[55] Hanne Elisabeth Dickmeiss conceded that differences of culture and mores made the evaluation of medical schools a continuing challenge. But the European schools with ties to schools in Britain were "embarrassingly close." She added that "Copenhagen, unrecognized, is as remote as Aberdeen, rather more ancient, uses English textbooks, and completes its anatomy courses in Glasgow. One of the leading characters at its foundation in 1479 was Alexander Kinghorn from Scotland, physician to King Kristain II."

Where *The Lancet* letters focused on the disparities produced by the registration machinery outside of Britain, those in the *British Medical Journal* were concerned with the presence of overseas doctors within Britain. Rather than symbolizing the best of British medicine, these letters argued, their presence reflected a highly distorted set of push and pull factors. To illustrate the role of personal gain in motivating overseas doctors, E. M. C. Allen selectively quoted from the response of the head of a radiology department in India to an advertisement for a British registrar position well below his level of experience: "A post in England would help me surmount the rigid foreign exchange restrictions imposed by the Reserve Bank of India."[56] Troubled, Allen added: "I also feel that perhaps the time has come to examine a little more closely our whole attitude towards postgraduate education of some of our overseas graduates if this [financial gain] is their aim and object."[57] For M. Sirajullah, it was not so much the motives of the doctors for "personal benefits" but the staffing needs of hospitals that transformed training posts into de facto career tracks. Hospitals preferred experienced doctors and were more inclined to renew their appointments to maintain staffing continuity and stability.[58] P. K. Chakrabarty reduced Allen's concern to a simple matter of supply and demand: "When the supply of British graduates meets the demands of British hospitals it will require very little 'examination' by Dr. Allen to stop our employment and training."[59]

The GMC did not respond to this rising tide of criticism about the registration of overseas doctors. This reflected the fact that the council was legally bound to follow the Medical Act and any attempt to change how overseas doctors were registered involved consulting with the council and the approval of the Privy Council. Ironically, this passive public posture invited other interests to weigh in and, in the process, increased attention to the disparate effects of registration for doctors with overseas qualifications. In August 1967 Ronald Gibson, the chairman of the council of the BMA, wrote to Lord Cohen requesting a meeting about Terrell's predicament.[60] In his meeting with Gibson as in his later presidential address to the council, Cohen did not make an affirmative argument on behalf of temporary registration; instead he stressed that the council had to work within the status quo.[61] While underscoring the council's statutory independence, this statement implicitly drew a distinction between the different realms of responsibility for overseas doctors in Britain—the council and the hospital hiring committees—while avoiding discussion of the national composition and linguistic and clinical competence of overseas doctors.

For Gibson and others, Terrell's case provided a vehicle to draw distinctions between the national origins and the capacity for belonging. Gibson's press release noted that "Mrs. Terrell has a Polish medical degree. From 1963 she worked here but her temporary registration with the General Medical Council stopped in 1965 when she married an English engineer." The facts—where she trained and marital status—pointed to Terrell's European origins and capacity for fitting into British society. Sir Cyril Black, a member of the House of Commons for Wimbledon and advocate for restrictions on new Commonwealth immigration, made the connection explicit when raising the matter on behalf of his constituent. Black pointed out her distinct advantage over unnamed Commonwealth countries: "She can speak, write and understand English."[62]

This was not the first time the question of the English-language competence of overseas doctors, particularly doctors from the Commonwealth, came up. In early 1966, the BMA General Medical Services Committee proposed the need for English-language testing for overseas doctors before entering into independent practice. Without comment, the BMA Council agreed and forwarded the recommendation to the General Medical Council. Although the recommendation referred to general practitioners, it was clear to at least one correspondent to the *British Medical Journal* that the implications for all overseas doctors in the hospital service would loom quite large. L. R. M. Kamal sought answers about the scope of overseas doctors envisaged by the recommendation. "Would the graduates from Australia, Canada, and New Zealand be required to face such an examination, or would it be specifically directed to graduates from India or Pakistan (they form the bulk of overseas graduates in this country, and their medium of instruction is English)? Would I, for that matter, after working in British hospitals for nearly four years, have to qualify in such an examination if I did not decide to enter into 'independent medical practice?'"[63]

Language Testing and Overseas Doctors: From Guidelines to Conditions of Employment (1967–71)

As the discussion about the Terrell case became more contentious, the health ministry approached the GMC about the registration of overseas-trained medical graduates. Seeking to prevent the registration controversy from complicating the amending legislation for the proposed retention fee, J. P. Cashman solicited the view of the GMC about a possible alternative route to full registration for doctors from nonreciprocating countries.[64] Their response consisted of two memoranda, reiterating the value of reciprocity as well as the existing paths to registration, temporary and full registration.[65] The first, prepared by registrar Walter Pykes-Lee, outlined the strength and limitations of existing arrangements of registration. The second, which summarized the views of Lord Cohen as president of the council alone, addressed provisions of the Medical Act that merited consideration for repeal or amendment.

Pyke-Lees framed temporary registration along with reciprocity as means to enhance the reputation of British medicine and project British influence in the world. He highlighted the significance of the temporary nature of the visit by invoking the metaphor of the United Kingdom as a *Medical Mecca*, a term attributed to the former secretary of the Medical Council of India. In place of an imperial relationship, medicine functioned as a voluntary means of sharing cultural identity across space and place. The visit was not so much about settlement, but a duty or "pilgrimage." During these visits, doctors simultaneously demonstrated their solidarity and submission to British medicine and returned home "fortified and illuminated" after having obtained hospital experience or an advanced qualification.[66]

Pyke-Lees was far more defensive about reciprocity. Unlike temporary registration, in which access to the medical market was a privilege bounded with restrictions, reciprocity granted admission to the register based on the presumptive equivalency of medical qualifications in reciprocating countries. He rejected the characterization of reciprocity by critics as an "instance of misplaced Victorian logic, irrelevant to the needs of the country."[67] Reciprocity reinforced the influence of Britain and British medicine in "old" and "new" Commonwealth countries that granted medical degrees. Rather than contracting with decolonization, Pyke-Lees anticipated further extensions "to cover more of the developing countries in the Commonwealth."[68] Countries like Ceylon, Burma, Malta, India, and Pakistan modeled their medical curriculum on the United Kingdom while the authority of the GMC to inspect schools for equivalency ensured consistency of standards. Far from seeing the authority as an imperial holdover, other countries actively sought the approval of the GMC for their national medical schools and qualifications as reflected in a report of a delegation from the GMC and the Privy Council to Burma. The report noted that the delegation was well received throughout their visit to Burma and left with the unmistakable impression that the local profession sought to strengthen the "long-standing links between Burmese and British medicine."[69] Given the underlying authority that reciprocity engendered, the council was skeptical about ending it. The special relationship that sustained the influence of the GMC in reciprocating countries would be placed in jeopardy. The training that foreign doctors obtained in the United Kingdom, the ability of the council to visit foreign medical schools, and the model of British medical education all would potentially be at risk or adversely impacted.[70]

While Pyke-Lees's memorandum largely affirmed the status quo, Lord Cohen elaborated on possible amendments to the Medical Act that might mitigate the restrictions associated with temporary registration.[71] A revision of the temporality language in section 25 appeared to be uncontroversial. The existing language tied the hands of the council even as it "tried to administer the requirement sympathetically" when advising foreign- and overseas-trained doctors.[72] In addition, the prescriptive nature of posts to be held and their scheduled termination had become too inflexible to accommodate "modern trends in medical practice, including specialist and vocational training." As much as Cohen believed that these restrictions were useful for doctors who were in need of postgraduate training, they needlessly imposed upon doctors seeking specialist training the need to continually renew their certificates. To correct this, Cohen floated the idea of expanding the authority of the council to determine the length of the period of temporary registration based on the nature of the specialty and duration of training necessary for competency or eligibility for higher qualifications.[73]

Although Lord Cohen was open to modifying the existing arrangements for temporary registration, he was far more hesitant to embrace substantial changes to the procedures for full registration. Contrary to press reports, foreign- and overseas-trained doctors appeared to make the most of requalification as a route to full registration. Commenting on the 568 doctors who requalified in a decade, Cohen observed that "these are not inconsiderable figures. They are far from confirming the pessimistic reports which have appeared in the press concerning the practicability of the procedure involved." At the same time, he conceded that the process for requalification was far from consistent among the three nonuniversity licensing bodies.[74] It was for these reasons that Cohen proposed consulting with these bodies to explore standardizing how the qualifications and experiences of foreign and overseas medical graduates were evaluated and who was permitted to sit for the various professional examinations leading to a British primary qualification.

As for the creation of a wholly new route to full registration that was disconnected from reciprocity, Cohen was noncommittal. It is likely that this would have involved more elaborate amending legislation, not to mention a potential change, if not increase, in workload for the council. Under the time constraints of the session of Parliament, this was impracticable. At the same time, Cohen outlined the conditions of an assessment regime. In so doing he straddled the reciprocity fence. On the one hand, the GMC had defended reciprocity rather warmly. On the other hand, obdurate resistance to even the consideration of an alternative route would have intensified criticism of the existing arrangements as arbitrary. At a minimum, this balancing act preserved the viability of reciprocity even though the suggested assessment regime for an alternative route in principle diluted it.

Cohen sketched a plan for a hybrid body charged with assessing the credentials and experience of foreign- and overseas-trained doctors who sought full registration. While a new body, its composition would reinforce the existing distribution of power within British medicine. Its composition would include representatives from the three nonuniversity licensing bodies and one representative from the GMC for the United Kingdom. The English Conjoint Board (Royal Colleges of Physicians and Surgeons of England), the Society of Apothecaries of England, and the Scottish Triple Qualification (Royal Colleges of Surgeons and Medicine, and Apothecaries of Scotland) would be responsible for administering the examinations for higher professional qualifications and would also enjoy institutional representation on the council. The components of the assessment would include confidential reports by consultants or senior members of the medical profession "which should be procured whenever possible from consultants in British hospitals on the performance of the applicant who have worked in those hospitals." Cohen emphasized three additional sources of information for scrutiny by the proposed assessment body: "(a) the standard of the original qualification of the applicant, (b) his professional experience outside this country (supporting documents would ordinarily be required), and (c) his knowledge of the English language." The body would forward these materials together with associated recommendations for registration to the GMC "with which it would grant full registration in cases considered to be suitable."[75] In short, this assessment regime would draw on the collective authority and institutional responsibility of the British medical establishment to determine if overseas doctors possessed the training and experience that was equivalent to a medical graduate of the United Kingdom for full registration.

While health ministry officials considered the suggestions of the GMC, Cohen initiated talks with representatives of the English Conjoint Board, the committee of management of the Scottish Triple Qualification, and the Society of Apothecaries of London. The talks yielded a uniform set of standards under which overseas doctors could be admitted to the final examination, thereby clarifying the path for full admission to the medical register. Under the proposed plan, representatives of the licensing bodies agreed on three paths by which overseas doctors could pursue full registration. Two principles governed the plan: (1) that overseas doctors possess qualifications recognized by the council and (2) that they be subject to uniform assessment expectations. For doctors with qualifications that entitled them to temporary registration automatically, they would be admitted to the final examination of any three of the licensing bodies after the completion of at least twelve months in an approved hospital and a testimonial that certified their professional skill, knowledge of English, and general suitability. The second path was designed with doctors like Victoria Terrell in mind. Temporarily registered doctors who intended to remain in Britain were no longer prohibited from pursuing full registration. Under the proposed plan, they now needed to present "evidence of satisfactory completion of a clinical attachment of 12 months' duration at a hospital approved by the body concerned." For all other overseas doctors whose qualifications were not recognized, the council would review their applications on a case-by-case basis "to see what exemptions, if any, might be granted on the basis of their previous training."[76]

This plan, which was adopted and implemented in early 1969, represented a new departure for the GMC. Language competence had never been a formal area that the council considered in terms of reviewing applications for temporary registration for overseas doctors. There was no reason to evaluate language competency. English had been the primary language of instruction in Indian medical schools during British rule and remained so after independence. If anything, attention to language competency was an incidental consideration that grew out of the interaction between the candidate for registration and representatives of the council. It was both a response to the growing public connection between clinical and language competence and an effort to restrict access to the medical market. The inclusion of English competence in a certificate of performance built on an existing feature of the clinical attachment scheme in the hospital service. This Ministry of Health–funded scheme provided overseas doctors with a monthlong orientation of the hospital service under the supervision of a senior member of the medical staff on a voluntary basis from 1966 to 1969. Thereafter, attachment became a condition of employment. Whether for registration or appointment in the hospital service, overseas doctors now faced a uniform expectation. But they did so without an explicit norm or objective basis for what constituted English-language competence. The certification of a senior member of the profession was thought to be sufficient.

These guidelines did little to quiet criticism. In truth, they were a supplement to the existing system of registration. Compulsory attachment for those seeking appointments in the hospital service applied only after overseas doctors were admitted to the register, not before. Nor was there any limitation on the unrestricted right to practice for overseas doctors with recognized qualifications from reciprocating countries. Some critics of the existing system wanted to condition registration on a common assessment for all doctors rather than just those who sought employment in the NHS.

The United States provided an alternative model.[77] Like Britain, the United States supplemented its domestic production of medical graduates with foreign medical graduates. This relationship only increased with the concurrent expansion of postwar health care and demand for medical labor. There was no national standardization of assessment because licensing was a state, rather than a federal, responsibility. The American Medical Association (AMA) attempted to exert its influence indirectly on state licensing boards by producing an annual list of approved foreign medical schools between 1950 and 1960. But, as Rosemary Stevens and Joan Vermeulen have discussed, it proved to be short-lived.[78] The inspection of medical schools was neither comprehensive nor consistently conducted. In place of attempting to appraise individual medical schools, a consortium of organizations, which included the AMA, the American Hospital Association, and the Federation of State Medical Boards, developed an examination for medical graduates. Administered by the Educational Council, the Foreign Medical Graduate Examination (ECFMGE) consisted of a multiple choice test of medical knowledge and an English-language test. Initiated in 1957, the examination was held semi-annually in the United States and at an expanding number of examination centers in 120 countries. It became a de facto condition of access to the profession due to a policy decision by the AMA. Its approval of hospital internship and residency programs was subject to foreign graduates either possessing a state license to practice or passing the ECFMGE.

The adoption of an ECFMG for Britain would have far-reaching implications for the GMC as well as the NHS. Temporary registration would cease to exist for all practical purposes. Along with the loss of critical fee revenue for the operations of the GMC, an important source of medical labor for the NHS would be less reliable, if not closed off altogether. More significantly, the imposition of an examination as a condition of entry for doctors with qualifications that entitled them to full registration would establish a double standard and contradict the spirit, if not the letter, of reciprocity. As noted by Pyke-Lees, the end of reciprocity would diminish the authority and power of the GMC to inspect and otherwise sustain British medicine as a worldwide standard. The preference of the GMC and the proposal of the BMA set up a political impasse whose solution would alter the place of overseas-trained doctors within British medicine.

Conclusion

Reflecting Britain's official postwar policy toward the Commonwealth, the GMC embraced globalization. Its system of overseas registration seamlessly managed the participation in the domestic medical market of doctors who received their primary qualification outside of the United Kingdom. The register simultaneously symbolized the global scope of British medicine and enabled Britain to harness the labor of doctors in support of the state's obligation under the NHS to delivery health care to the public as a right of citizenship. Yet the global reach of British medicine and the system of registration itself became a site of scrutiny as tensions between the profession and the government about pay and conditions mounted. The discourses associated with the movements both of domestic medical graduates to the "old" Commonwealth and of the doctors from the United States and "new" Commonwealth countries to the United Kingdom recast membership in British medicine in terms that privileged whiteness and Europeanness at the expense of the nonwhite Commonwealth. For critics of the system of overseas registration, the status of reciprocating and nonreciprocating countries distorted the social structure of British medicine. The rigid restrictions associated with temporary registration deprived the NHS of qualified doctors from European countries. Conversely, the entitlement to full registration enjoyed by nonwhite doctors exposed the public to doctors whose priorities and cultural difference were deemed inadequate to, if not incompatible with, British medicine.

The rapidity with which the system of overseas registration became a liability not only reflected the GMC's institutional vulnerability, but also informed how it responded. The 1886 Medical Acts and its amendments charged the GMC to oversee registration to minimize the impact of overseas doctors on the domestic profession. In practice, its authority was circumscribed by either a permissive system of full registration based on reciprocity or a rigid set of conditions as provided for temporary registration. These sources of trained medical professionals supplemented the historically flat domestic production of medical graduates without impacting medical schools or the profession at large. If anything, the fees associated with their registration masked the financial insecurity of the GMC while minimizing fee increases for domestic medical graduates. The success of the globalization of the register—namely, projecting British medicine in the world, accessing trained medical labor, and delivering heath care to the nation—opened up the GMC to criticism that it was failing to police the social boundaries of British medicine. No event better illustrated the politics of overseas registration than that involving Victoria Terrell. Even though the GMC enforced the provisions of the 1948 Medical Act in prohibiting the extension of her temporary registration, Terrell's supporters and critics of reciprocity portrayed the system of registration as obsolete, one that diluted British medicine by preferentially treating overseas doctors from "new" Commonwealth countries over European countries.

For its part, the council defended the value of overseas registration to Britain as well as its administration of the register. Bound by legislative mandate, it could not do otherwise. Validating the discourse about the competency of overseas doctors also ran the risk of alienating an important source of revenue. But its defense would prove to be contingent. Seeking to stabilize its financial affairs, the council in 1968 secured approval from the Privy Council for an annual retention fee for all doctors to remain on the British register. This shift in subsidizing the GMC from one that was dependent on overseas doctors to one based on the contributions of domestic doctors simultaneously increased the profession's scrutiny of the GMC and the council's attention to the processes of overseas registration.

Chapter Six

Managing the Political Problem of the Registration of Overseas Doctors, 1971–73

Introduction

As the place of overseas doctors became politically contentious within and outside of the medical profession, the liminal place of the GMC between the state and the profession made it highly sensitive to political pressure. To be sure, the council possessed regulatory authority. But the effective power of the GMC was minimized by its constitutional subordination to the Privy Council, not to mention the government's legislative mandates. Its capacity for independent action was diluted further by the autonomy of university and nonuniversity licensing bodies, which comprised the majority of the representatives on the council. Nonuniversity licensing bodies, for example, were able to use their own discretion in determining whether the conditions for requalification had been met by overseas candidates, relying on their expertise in assessing candidates' professional experience.

Furthermore, the virtual absence of supplementary sources of funding curbed the GMC's capacity for pursuing independent initiatives. Until the establishment of the category of temporary registration for overseas doctors, the GMC had maintained a hand-to-mouth existence. To subsidize its operations, the GMC relied on the one-time fee for life paid by domestic medical graduates who were admitted to the register to subsidize its operations. Fees from overseas doctors proved advantageous in the short run but were not a permanent solution to financial stability as hostility against nonwhite Commonwealth immigration grew. Indeed, one unintended consequence of the 1962 Commonwealth Immigration Act, which mandated work vouchers for all Commonwealth immigrants, was the drop in the number of overseas doctors seeking admission to the register. As costs associated with the operation of the GMC continued to climb, this reduction of revenue spurred the council to look to the domestic medical profession for a more reliable source of support.

The development of a more regular source of revenue would produce a trade-off for the GMC: financial security heightened scrutiny from organized medicine. In 1966 the council proposed a new retention fee. Instead of a one-time fee for life, all doctors would now be required to pay an annual fee to remain on the register and continue to be legally entitled to practice medicine. Preferring an independent body to one dependent on state support, the British Medical Association (BMA) council agreed to the fee despite opposition from its membership. The effect of the fee, which was enacted in 1971 after passage of the 1969 Medical Act, was not politically neutral. On the contrary, in diminishing the GMC's dependency on overseas doctors for revenue, it increased the leverage of the association. As resentment and resistance within the membership increased, the BMA advised its members to condition their payment of the fee on a review of the GMC's budget. They also pressed for changes in the regulation of the medical profession, which had been in development for several years. The BMA not only insisted on expanding the composition of the council to include a majority of directly elected members from the profession at large, but also called for a major overhaul of overseas registration. Their newly proposed system promised to recast the territorial and social boundaries of British medicine. Reciprocity was to be eliminated and the number of routes to the register reduced to only one. All candidates for temporary registration would be required to pass a language and professional assessment examination. In truth, the association's proposal did not seek to end the globalization of British medicine. But in limiting the domestic impact of globalization to temporary trained labor, the register would formalize two tiers of the medical profession: those who were trained in Britain and those who were not. These tiers would effectively codify racial difference within the profession based on national origins.

The council leadership began redefining the relationship of overseas doctors to British medicine within its existing authority. It appointed a special committee and charged it to make recommendations. The committee's report retroactively defended the integrity of the system of overseas registration but acknowledged the need for changes in light of the worldwide proliferation of medical schools and the decline of English as the cultural glue of British medicine in "new" Commonwealth countries. The recommendations included the creation of a dedicated committee tasked with overseeing overseas doctors. The existence of this committee would simultaneously underscore the perceived problem of overseas doctors within British medicine and their difference from domestic medical graduates. Still another recommendation called for testing all candidates for temporary registration. This latter recommendation reinforced the suspicion about the clinical and cultural competency of overseas doctors. As this chapter will show, the GMC and BMA would find far more consensus on reforming the system of overseas registration than on other issues.

The GMC and the Pursuit of Financial Stability, 1965–69

Until 1963, the fees from overseas doctors, which supplemented the revenue from domestic medical graduates, masked the GMC's hand-to-mouth existence. But inflation drove up the basic costs of running the council, ranging from labor and national insurance contribution to heating. The one elastic source of revenue, registration fees from overseas doctors, became imperiled by domestic politics. The passage of the Commonwealth Immigration Act in 1962 signaled the redefinition of British nationality. The right of citizens from Commonwealth countries to work in the United Kingdom was curbed. In the wake of race riots in 1958, the provision that migrants possess a voucher from an employer before entering the county to work functioned to check the flow of nonwhite immigrants to the United Kingdom.[1] One immediate impact of the act was a drop in overseas doctors seeking admission to the register. Even though the legislation actually provided exemptions for doctors, advertising this would have blunted the political message of the bill. The drop in revenue after the implementation of the act both exposed the fragility of the financial position of the GMC and spurred the council to find more permanent funding alternatives.

The options available to the council were limited. Supplementing or replacing fees with government support was one possibility. But this would undermine the council's statutory independence and create the impression that it was an agency of the state. The only viable options that guaranteed its independence while meeting its current year revenue needs involved raising existing fees or imposing new fees on domestic medical graduates on the register. It is a measure of the council's desperation that President Cohen approached the Privy Council in 1964 for authorization to raise registration fees to six pounds for provisional and twelve pounds for full registration. This request was part of a two-step request. The increase for existing fees was to apply to the 1965 fiscal year. The council also requested authorization to introduce a new annual two-pound retention fee for doctors already on the medical register and a reduction of the fees for provisional and full registration to four pounds and six pounds respectively.

The proposed retention fee represented a major change in the fee structure for doctors and to the revenue stream for the GMC. Since the establishment of the medical register in 1858, doctors had always paid a one-time fee for lifetime admission to the registration.[2] Although the retention fee would be tax deductible, the culminated costs for a doctor during a projected forty-year career would increase more than four times: from twenty-one pounds to ninety pounds.[3] The proposed fee structure in effect shifted the costs for the operations of the GMC to all doctors and not just new doctors admitted to the register. The projected revenue was estimated to yield several hundred thousand pounds annually from this one source alone. This, combined with temporary registration fees, would allow the GMC to achieve financial stability. However, proposing and implementing the retention fee were two difference propositions. As an additional condition to practice medicine legally in Britain, the proposed retention fee would require an amendment to the Medical Acts. This involved persuading the government to introduce such legislation while consulting with relevant government departments and turning to organizations within the medical profession for support. Of the latter, the support of the BMA was particularly important in light of the fact that it represented by far the largest number of doctors to be affected by the proposed fee.

The rationale given for the retention fee was grounded in the importance of preserving the independence of the GMC while ensuring the execution of its duties. But the need to shift the burden to domestic medical graduates, who were the overwhelming majority on the register, was rendered in narrowly national terms by representing overseas doctors as an unreliable source of income. In reference to operating deficits between 1950 and 1961, the proposal acknowledged that "the Council was able to avoid these deficits in most of these years as a result of remarkable increases in the number of Commonwealth and foreign doctors who applied for registration." Obliquely alluding to the impact of the Commonwealth Immigration Act, the report continued, "In 1962, however, as a result of political and economic factors entirely outside of the Council's control, the total abruptly fell to 26,300 pounds and the decline continued in 1963. As the Council's expenses continued to increase in these years, the results were heavy deficits."[4] Such declines in applicant fees in the early 1960s "afforded no secure financial basis for the work of a statutory body charged with responsibilities as those of the Council in the fields of medical education, registration, and discipline."[5] This characterization not only implied that British doctors carried a special obligation to subsidize the function of the GMC for the future but also masked the high registration fees for doctors who qualified outside of the Commonwealth. Depending on the length of the period of temporary registration, they ranged from three pounds, ten shillings for up to two months to ten pounds in excess of two months. These fees were greater than the proposed retention fee or equivalent for provisional and full registration.

The response to the retention fee was one of resigned acceptance among the leadership of the association. The BMA Council, in principle, accepted the rationale for the fee.[6] An editorial in the *British Medical Journal* reached the same conclusion. "Against a background of continual inflation the once-for-all fee is an anachronism; it condemns the newly qualified practitioners to bearing the whole burden of rising costs, which is clearly unfair. Annual fees seem inescapable, but their level will always need to be watched closely."[7] Yet the rationale for shifting the costs associated with the regulation of the profession reinforced, rather than minimized, differences between domestic and overseas graduates. The financial lifeline of the retention fee took place in a context in which the presence of overseas doctors in British medicine in general and in the hospital service in particular had become highly politicized, so much so that the Ministry of Health in 1965 introduced the clinical attachment scheme to supervise and assess registered overseas doctors before they entered into their hospital appointments.

The Clinical Attachment Scheme and the Politics of Competency

Doubts about the competency of overseas-trained doctors were framed initially in terms of the reputation of the training provided in the United Kingdom. "What worried responsible commentators," a leader in the *British Medical Journal* volunteered, "is the fact that the young doctors from abroad have found many British hospitals ill-equipped to give them the post-graduate training which so many of them come to seek."[8] Robin Burkitt warned that such conditions jeopardized the credibility of British medicine in the world. Overseas doctors might "scrape through examination and return home possessed with the diploma but with none of the rooted knowledge which possession of the diploma is believed to imply. They will then take posts necessitating a clinical responsibility for which they are quite unfitted, and the teaching which they give will perpetuate false dogmas which they have never had the opportunity of disproving in the light of their experience."[9] This view was echoed by the 1961 Working Party on Medical Aid to Developing Countries, which was tasked to propose ways "to work out a coherent and coordinated response to the challenge presented by the medical needs of the developing world." In their final report, the group called for more rather than less supervision and assessment of overseas doctors. It strongly endorsed an attachment scheme proposed by H. W. Hutton, the overseas officer of the Royal College of Physicians.

Under Hutton's plan, two overseas graduates would be assigned to a consultant or a regional consultant group for two months. During this period, they would complete a rotation of the principal hospital departments and take case histories and performance procedures under the watchful eyes of their consultant. At the completion of the attachment period, the consultant would provide a certificate or testimonial for hospital boards that translated the participant's overseas education and training into the appropriate appointment grade in the service. A joint proposal between the University of Birmingham and the Birmingham Regional Hospital Board piloted Hutton's plan with a three-year grant from the Nuffield Trust. This pilot program fleshed out some of the content of the curriculum, including tutorials in the almoner's service, medico-legal procedures, and the English language. Despite the high expectations of the organizers, the program was declared all but a failure within a year. Two more cohorts followed with little improvement. A. G. W. Whitefield and A. J. McCall linked the failure of the program to a mismatch between the program assumptions and the actual preferences of overseas doctors. They noted that "a considerable proportion do not wish to hold house officer appointments, and many of those who take them do so merely as a means of paying their way while they are reading for higher examination—not for the clinical and educational opportunities the appointment provides." They proposed changes to align preferences with attachment. These included the provision of a stipend and conditioning house officer appointment and effective eligibility for higher examinations on the completion of a six-to-eight-week period of training and assessment.[10]

Even though the pilot program proved to be ineffectual, the Health Ministry adopted the Commonwealth School model in 1965. It is difficult not to see this decision as a gesture to mitigate political damage to the hospital service and the government. There was really no practical solution that could rebut the growing skepticism about overseas doctors. Attachment provided a tool for reconciling the politically contentious paradox of the hospital service, a national service that was dependent on largely nonwhite overseas doctors. In theory the oversight by white male senior medical professionals symbolized a quality control safeguard. They would ensure that overseas doctors understood how to navigate the NHS and were equipped to practice medicine in a clinical setting. In this role, senior doctors served as cultural gatekeepers as much as guides to the structure of the career. Their assessment of attached doctors included English-language competency. But in the absence of any objective standard or norm, the credibility of the assessment—and, by extension, public confidence—reflected a highly subjective notion of the facility of the English language.

Internally, the government moved to mandate attachment as a condition of employment for hospital appointments as early as 1966. But this condition would not go into effect until 1969. In the meantime, there were too few points of control when qualified doctors needed employment and hospital hiring boards needed to fill vacancies. Health Ministry officials felt that too few doctors were volunteering for attachment and that the participation of those who did was inconsistent. Out of the 844 applicants in 1966, 372 attachments were offered and only 119 certificates of completion were issued. "It is particularly disturbing that up to one third of those reporting for attachment are found to be deficient in either clinical competence or command of English." M. R. P. Grogson wrote in justification of the change to mandatory attachment training: "This is of concern both as regards those who complete attachment and for its implications as regards the much larger number who do not, but obtain employment (often in the Senior House Office grade) without previous experience in this country."[11] The ministry deferred implementing the change until 1969 to give hospitals time to coordinate and to secure the cooperation of consultants. In the meantime, participation remained low while official concerns about language competency persisted. In a memorandum for the cabinet committee on immigration and community relations, L. G. Morgan of the Department of Employment and Productivity pointed out that

> even though Commonwealth doctors, although their undergraduate course in medicine was given in English, may find difficulty in understanding colloquial English and in making themselves readily understood by patients. A good grasp of colloquial English is especially important for doctors in accident and emergency departments. Ability to communicate with patients is an important factor in determining whether a doctor is suitable for a particular post and hospital authorities have been asked to ensure that their arrangements for selecting doctors for employment take this into account.[12]

The British Medical Association was openly skeptical of attachment. They preferred assessing doctors before they were admitted to the register, not after. At the twelfth annual clinical meeting of the BMA on the island of Malta in early 1969, the overseas affairs committee proposed replacing attachment altogether with more stringent conditions for admission to the register. These included restricting admission to candidates who were eligible for full registration and passed an English-language competency test.[13] A *BMJ* editorial tied the committee's recommendations to a perverse set of incentives and disincentives that had produced the current crisis in British medicine. "The existing situation—a rising pool of unemployed overseas doctors and a widening gulf between jobs which are worth while and those that can be filled only from the unemployed—should not be allowed to deteriorate." The constrained choice of hospital hiring boards, like the decision of domestic medical graduates to migrate, exposed and exacerbated disparities in health care resources in the United Kingdom. The editorial remarked that "a consultant in a northern-mill-town is often faced with the choice of no houseman or one with no previous experience in Britain and with poor command of English. Should he take on such a candidate, hoping to find him a useful pair of hands while he learns English? Whose responsibility is it if a tragedy occurs because of misunderstanding or failure in communications."[14] This pointed reference to government culpability echoed the committee's call for an immediate meeting between representatives of the association, the relevant government offices, and the GMC to address the crisis. Secretary of State for Health and Social Services Richard Crossman agreed to meet in March.

In preparing a briefing document for Crossman, senior DHSS personnel explored the implications of the BMA proposal.[15] The proposal was consequential insofar as it would require amending the Medical Acts to authorize the GMC to impose a language test on all applicants trained overseas, regardless of whether they were from a reciprocating country. This test placed reciprocity at risk. It constituted an additional requirement or condition for registration that other countries did not impose on British medical graduates. Logically, doctors who failed the test would lose their right of appeal to the Privy Council.[16] There were wider political implications to the effective termination of reciprocity. There was likely to be possible accusations of selective discrimination, if not resentment, among major donor countries such as India and Pakistan. This outcome ran the risk of straining intragovernment relations. It was assumed that the Foreign and Commonwealth Office regarded reciprocity as a means to promote British influence in the Commonwealth, particularly among university-educated members of the professional classes.[17]

At the same time, there was concern that such a language examination would complicate Britain's early entry negotiations with the European Economic Community (EEC) as it related to the mutual recognition of medical qualifications.[18] After two previous attempts in 1963 and 1967, Britain's application would be accepted in 1971. But being outside and looking in on the EEC since 1950 limited Britain's capacity to shape community-wide policies, especially concerning the recognition of medical qualifications. Under a draft directive of the EEC, doctors from member countries would undergo a six-month period of adaptation, which functioned loosely like clinical attachment. As senior DHSS personnel noted in their briefing documents, the adaptation period was an administrative requirement, not a condition of registration per se. It was to "ensure that the doctors wishing to practice in a country other than their own had adequate mastery of the language, customs and the health and social legislation (in particular the social security system)." But there was no expectation that "any one would 'fail.'" There was concern in Britain that any implementation of a language requirement would backfire. "It therefore seems clear that writing a linguistic qualification into the Medical Act would lead to international criticism and cause particular difficulties should entry into Europe become an immediate possibility."[19]

Furthermore, the effect of the proposed changes would require a significant modification in the workload of the GMC. The expectation of language competence for overseas doctors who sought full registration through requalification was a recent development. Up until this point, the council's oversight was not direct, since the testimonial of a senior member of the medical staff certified competence. In light of the twenty countries of origin of applicants seeking temporary registration certificates in 1968, the implementation of a language examination presented logistical and financial challenges for an organization that lacked experience and already struggled with operating budget deficits. Nor was there an obvious alternative to the GMC. While taking the examination in Britain would be easier than doing so abroad, there were related problems. Given the scale of the applicants for temporary registration in the recent past, the administration of an examination would require considerable staffing and space. There was also the not insignificant matter of financial responsibility: "Cost might be a problem—the G.M.C. would not want to pay for the examination system itself and would not accept a grant, and there might be difficult in securing sufficient fee income from the applicants." A related issue added a further complication: the financial exigency of applicants who failed the examination. "It might well be necessary to provide money for their return, and perhaps even to provide English courses."[20]

Although it was within the authority of the government to move legislation to amend the Medical Act "to require the G.M.C. to register and test the qualifications of immigrant doctors," Crossman did not seek such legislation. Judging from his cabinet diary, he was unafraid of the political fallout. What made such a course problematic was pending legislation before the House of Commons to amend the Medical Act. The proposed legislation provided for two changes for which there appeared to be a consensus. One authorized the GMC to impose a retention fee on all registered doctors and the second repealed the length of stay clause, thereby permitting overseas doctors with temporary registration certificates to seek full registration via requalification. Crossman recalled that "the papers had come to me to say that the Department had looked into this [the implementation of a language examination] and found no necessity for it and they wanted the non-controversial Bill to go to the Legislation Committee at once."[21] The decision to go forward with the bill as proposed meant that mandating an English-language competency examination would remain a possibility for the future. In the meantime, the ministry was left with one existing tool to manage overseas doctors: the clinical attachment scheme. Crossman proposed making attachment compulsory as an alternative to language testing. "The only difficulty with that," he commented, "is that we need so many immigrant doctors each year that there aren't enough consultants to give them the month's attachment."[22]

Britain's reliance on overseas doctors was accepted as a basic condition for the foreseeable future. For this reason, Crossman solicited the views of the BMA only regarding the "quantity" and "quality" of overseas-trained doctors, not regarding whether they should practice medicine at all in the United Kingdom.[23] Underlying this formulation was not only a distinction between those trained inside and outside of the United Kingdom, but also the political imperative to improve the oversight of overseas doctors before they were admitted to the register. The discussion of temporary registration formed part of a wider discussion of the perceived weaknesses in managing access to the British labor market after 1961. The voucher program set quotas on the number of skilled workers entering the country to work while the system of temporary registration regulated access to the medical market. The voucher program mandated that all non–UK resident citizens apply for and receive a voucher as a condition to work legally in Britain. Medical professionals received a higher proportion of Category "B" vouchers, which referred to preferred skills that the country needed. But critics in the profession accused hospitals of circumventing the application process by appointing overseas doctors, who were in Britain on a travel or study visa, and thereafter requesting an emergency voucher from the Home Office. Rather than conceding the abuse by hiring authorities, Crossman was prepared to consider preferential treatment for doctors: "Doctors ought not to be discriminated against in immigration control; but it is for consideration whether it is right to continue to discriminate in their favor as in the past." To this end, he pledged that he would "keep continuous watch on the figures and would not hesitate to propose action to prevent it rising much above 1,000 a year if necessary." Beyond this point, the department was loath to do more than make refinements to the voucher program.[24]

While "quantity" was defined in terms of the operation of the voucher program, the discussion about temporary registration was framed as a problem of assessing "quality."[25] Although the GMC based its decisions on the credentials and experience of overseas applicants for registration, this was "no guarantee that a doctor's command of English is adequate for the particular work he has to do." The GMC had even less control when it came to overseas doctors with recognized medical qualifications from reciprocating counties. "The G.M.C. can take knowledge of English into account in relation to aliens who seek temporary registration for a specific post, but doctors from the Commonwealth are entitled to registration, if they are from a recognized school, without any such test." More so than the GMC, the hospitals as hiring authorities had the "duty" to ensure that "the doctors they appoint have a sufficient command of the English language for the work they have to do." But this proved to be insufficient, and it was "disturbing that criticisms are still being made about the minority of overseas doctors who have difficulty in making themselves understood." Crossman invited suggestions about how knowledge of English might be tested and in what ways doctors should be helped to improve their communication skills. Still another area where the profession's input was needed was in making clinical attachment a condition of employment in the hospital service rather than voluntary.[26]

The March 20 meeting included key personnel, including Crossman and Under-Secretary of State Alfred Bavin, Assistant Secretary A. Gilmour, Chief Medical Officer George Godber, GMC president Lord Cohen, BMA chair Ronald Gibson, Secretary D. Stevenson, and Deputy-Chairman of the Central Committee for Hospital Medical Services R. Mayne-White. As the briefing paper outlined, the meeting was designed to solicit input from the association, not to determine policy. There was broad agreement that the English-language competency of overseas doctors had become a problem that required corrective intervention. But the principals were divided about means. Alluding to the openness of Lord Cohen, Crossman stated that he was prepared to explore the "feasibility of English language assessment," but little more, and he was certainly not willing to amend legislation. The association had a definite view about the function of language testing. Its priority was to narrow access to the medical market by linking language testing to registration. This approach had the advantage of preserving reciprocal relations while discouraging overseas doctors from coming to Britain on a travel visa and seeking emergency vouchers. Representatives of the BMA agreed in principle with language testing as a condition of employment, preferring the administration of any test in the country of primary qualification.[27]

The consultation with the medical profession did not yield new legislation during the remaining year and a half of the Labor government. The noncontroversial bill became law in July 1969. But the question of language testing did not go away. The *BMJ* commented on the lacuna in the bill that passed: "Many people . . . [saw] the Medical Bill as an opportunity for putting a language test on a more formal basis, presumably by making command of English a condition of registration."[28] Little changed when it came to regulating the access of overseas doctors to the British medical market. The conditions for temporary and full registration remained unchanged, though the amended Medical Act repealed language in section 25 that required applicants to pledge their intention to leave the United Kingdom once their scheduled period of registration ended. Still, doctors with recognized medical qualifications from reciprocating countries were entitled to automatic registration without consideration of their language ability or additional assessment with regard to their clinical competence. It is likely that the council scrutinized in-person applicants for temporary registration about their English language. The voucher program remained in place, though the government pledged to cap the total number. It is likely that hospitals, in need of medical staff, and overseas doctors, in need of training and a regular income, continued to circumvent the voucher application process. While compulsory attachment as a condition of appointment in the hospital service marked a new departure, the BMA and GMC viewed it as too little too late.

Nevertheless, a significant development was achieved before the Conservative Party assumed the levers of government: a consensus on the necessity for assessing the language competency of overseas doctors. The association had pressed the issue since the 1960s and the GMC had listened. Following up on its proposal to harmonize the guidelines for requalification as outlined in the GMC memorandum to the Department of Health, the council introduced English competency as one of the criteria. Admittedly, the numbers of such cases were small in comparison to other registration categories. These guidelines demonstrated how the council would use its authority to address pressing problems. In the absence of the repeal of reciprocity, the GMC and the government would pursue other means to achieve this end. In the meantime, the GMC initiated the development of a test that was to determine who was fit to practice British medicine.

GMC Special Committee on Registration of Overseas Doctors, 1972

Lord Cohen as president of the GMC defended the system of registration for overseas doctors, but this did not mean he was not open to public criticism of the system. In February 1971, the council directed the executive and registration committees to consider whether an internal review of arrangements for overseas doctors was warranted.[29] The appointment of a special committee amounted to an acknowledgment that overseas doctors were seen as a problem for British medicine. At the same time, the proposed review provided the council with a political space to engage in more of an active, rather than a reactive, role in shaping the conditions under which overseas doctors in the future would be entitled to practice medicine in Britain. The charge of the special committee was broad: to review "the present arrangements for the registration in this country of doctors who have qualified overseas, with a view to determining whether those arrangements are satisfactory and, insofar as they are unsatisfactory, to make recommendations for changes in time."[30] In this capacity, the committee, which consulted with professional organizations in the United Kingdom and Commonwealth and received written evidence, defined the scope of the problem and proposed a solution. To this end, the committee scrutinized allegations about the deficiencies of overseas doctors, evaluated complaints about the disparate impact of the system of registration for doctors trained within and outside of the Commonwealth, and considered alternative methods for assessing linguistic competence for registration applications.

Within a year of soliciting and considering evidence, the committee produced an interim report. Authored by Cohen, the report consisted of a summary of the evidence and proposed new arrangements. Cohen first turned to allegations about the clinical and linguistic competency of overseas doctors. Addressing these allegations was important to buttress public confidence in patient care and the credibility of the oversight of the council. The evaluation relied on the assessor reports for the clinical attachment scheme. Unlike anecdotal accounts that could not be confirmed, these assessments possessed the virtue of reflecting the opinion of a senior member of the medical profession who supervised the participating doctors over three months. The committee found little support for allegations of professional incompetence: "In the majority of cases in which unsatisfactory reports were received the adverse comment was on proficiency in English rather than on clinical competence, although in a few cases the doctor was deemed unsatisfactory on both grounds." While not an explicit rebuttal to criticism, this finding conveyed the sense that the council had been effective in its oversight: "On the evidence before it the Committee is bound to conclude that very few overseas doctors have so far been deficient."[31]

The committee was far more concerned about the linguistic capacity of overseas doctors in the future. While the report did acknowledge concerns about the communication skills of overseas doctors, it qualified them by emphasizing the special challenge of local dialects.[32] Implied in the attention to language competency was the centrality of English language as fundamental to the cultural integrity of British medicine and no less to the Commonwealth. As the empire shrunk rapidly after the war, English became an even more important marker of belonging in Britain. At the same time, in former British colonies the politics of decolonization had marked English as a language of alien rule, encouraging instead the reclamation of indigenous languages as part of the process of liberation and the formation of new national identities. Medicine was one of the few areas where English remained the primary language of instruction in successor states of the empire. Its privileged place reflected the historically dominant role of British doctors and texts in medical education in the empire.

Since these ties were a product of the historical enmeshment of British medicine in the imperial project, however, they were not unaffected by the end of empire. Based on trends in medical education, the committee forecast more challenges in preserving the recognized standard of British medicine while admitting medical personnel who received their primary medical training outside of the United Kingdom. The proliferation of medical schools made it difficult to ensure that this standard of medical education could be maintained over time for full or temporary registration qualifications. The committee continued, "Secondly, the increasing replacement of English by national languages in many countries is such that language difficulties are likely to increase in the future, even if English is retained as the official language of instruction in their Medical Schools."[33]

Among those giving evidence, opinion about the utility of reciprocity as safeguard was mixed at best. For most, it had become obsolete. Rather than a bulwark for British medicine throughout the Commonwealth, the Scottish Home and Health Department viewed it as contributing to the lack of confidence in competency. It called for a narrower definition of standards that served Britain while leaving other countries to set their own.[34] Others entertained a more qualified view about reciprocal arrangements for registration. For the British Postgraduate Medical Federation, the Council of the BMA, and the Department of Health and Social Sciences, reciprocity could still serve as a viable tool to regulate the transnational movement of doctors with either special skills or those who sought them, provided that the council could satisfy themselves as to the standards of their medical schools.[35]

Opinion was just as mixed for introducing English-language testing. In its letter, the Royal College of Physicians and Surgeons of Glasgow regarded language difficulties as due to variations in dialect rather than comprehension.[36] By contrast, the Society of Apothecaries of London endorsed testing, as did the British Medical Association. The council of the BMA noted that "serious problems arise from time to time from language difficulties, and that some kind of language test should undoubtedly be included on the assessment of the overseas applicant for registration."[37] Yet the responsibility for and reliability of language testing was another matter. The Royal College of Physicians and Surgeons of Glasgow, the Royal College of Physicians of England, and the Scottish Home and Health Department deemed such testing as outside the competence of the council and a responsibility that rested with the employing authority. The British Postgraduate Medical Federation raised doubts about the appropriateness of a general test to assess doctors who may be in a variety of posts and clinical situations.[38]

The Scottish Council for Postgraduate Medical Education represented a minority view in calling for replacing the recognition of qualifications with individual assessment. The council recommended that all overseas doctors undergo clinical and linguistic assessment administered by the main professional bodies—the English Conjoint Board in England and the Triple Qualification Board in Scotland. Passage would be a precondition for a limited registration and only for appointment in an approved NHS hospital. This proposal resembled the model of the United States Educational Council Foreign Medical Graduates Examination (ECFMGE), which had surfaced from time to time in the medical press. Set in the country of primary qualification or at least outside Britain, the examination would narrow the portal of entry into the medical market while providing a definitive determination about the competency of the overseas doctor to practice medicine. The level of interest in the examination and its role in the registration process varied.

Some, such as the Council of Postgraduate Medical Education in England and the British Postgraduate Medical Federation, endorsed the idea but remained convinced that inspection of medical schools as a condition of recognition for reciprocating countries was still possible or that exceptions should be provided for graduates of medical schools in North America. The council of the BMA was no less mixed in its response, though they still recommended some form of assessment as a condition of limited registration. The Department of Health and Social Security, for example, suggested several alternative forms of assessment, including successful completion of clinical attachment unless exempted, a pass on the USFMG examination, or obtaining a qualification recognized for temporary registration exclusively.[39]

In Cohen's presentation of the findings of the special committee, he highlighted the difficulties associated with adopting an ECFMG-style examination. These chiefly referred to the place of Britain and British medicine in the Commonwealth and wider world. Unlike the US government, which sponsored the examination in countries throughout the world, the British Department of Health was not forthcoming with such support. In addition, the willingness of other countries to host the examination was by no means a foregone conclusion. Alluding to India and Pakistan among others, Cohen observed that "a number of countries from whom overseas doctors now come to this country in significant numbers have refused to permit the holding of such an examination on their territory." Quite apart from undermining relations within the Commonwealth and jeopardizing the supply of overseas doctors, such an examination might introduce a complication in Britain's undertakings as it sought to join the EEC.[40]

Rather than resolving the tension between registration and assessment, the clinical attachment scheme highlighted them. Much of the criticism directed at the special committee about the scheme was not new. It included concerns about an imbalance between the supply of and the demand for slots, high rates of incompletion and insufficient consequences for unsatisfactory assessments, and mismatches in specialty fields between assessors and overseas doctors. The Royal College of Obstetricians and Gynaecologists and the Scottish Council for Postgraduate Education doubted the effectiveness of the attachment program in assessing doctors' facility to speak English. The Hospital Junior Staff Group Council viewed attachment as wholly flawed, while others, such as the Council of Postgraduate Education in England and Wales, thought it could be improved upon. The Royal College of Physicians and Surgeons of Glasgow viewed it favorably but suggested reducing the length of observation to one week.[41]

The special committee endorsed the continuation of the council's recognition of primary qualifications as the chief mode of assessment. At the same time, the committee was not indifferent to concerns about safeguarding medical standards while ensuring access to the medical market. To this end, the report recommended (without providing details) that clinical attachment be strengthened. More significantly, the privileged position of overseas doctors from reciprocating Commonwealth countries would be diluted. The special committee proposed ending reciprocity as a condition for full registration for overseas doctors. This was associated with the creation of a new registration category. Temporary registration was to be abolished and replaced with limited registration. Limited registration gave the council latitude in designating a wider range of appointments for open-ended periods. These features would reduce the administrative costs of tracking overseas doctors and lowered their need for costly renewals. Provision was also made for overseas doctors to proceed from limited to full registration after satisfactory service, to sit for the final professional examination and thereby be eligible for full registration. Finally, provisional registration was limited to graduates of the United Kingdom. Overseas doctors would have to complete their preregistration training in the countries of primary qualification.[42]

Cohen invited and received comments on the interim report from governmental and national medical bodies through the summer. He hoped for a consensus on the proposed arrangements for the registration of overseas doctors before submitting the final report to the full council for approval by November 1972. This sequence of consultation was prudent insofar as the proposed changes would involve several amendments to the existing medical act and as such would require the endorsement of both the Privy Council and the parliamentary Bills Committee for consideration in the current session. The Department of Health and Social Sciences regarded the proposed new arrangements favorably.[43] They ensured an uninterrupted supply of qualified personnel for the health service while preserving public confidence in medical standards. Noting that another decade or more would pass before Britain could be self-sufficient in its domestic supply of medical graduates, a memo summarized the department's position: "It is therefore highly important that any revision of the arrangements for recognition of overseas medical qualifications should not present unnecessary obstacles in the way of doctors from overseas wishing to work here whose qualifications meet UK requirements."[44]

Other responses to the special council report challenged key elements of the proposals, namely the role of the GMC in the recognition of primary degrees and the additional route to full registration for doctors from nonreciprocating countries. The BMA council welcomed the movement away from reciprocity. After considering the report further, the council offered two additional proposals. The first restricted registration only to overseas doctors who were eligible for full registration, "overseas doctors of high repute and distinction who are accredited by a Royal College or specialist faculty." The second proposed shifting responsibility for all other overseas doctors from the GMC to the nonuniversity medical bodies, which would assess the candidates' clinical and linguistic competency. Those who successfully passed the examination would be required to complete a one-year probationary period, "in the same way as a U.K. graduate is required to undergo a pre-registration year after primary qualification."[45]

The Scottish Council for Postgraduate Medical Education was by far the most searching in its criticism of the proposed category of limited registration.[46] Without an expectation of postgraduate training, there was a real risk of creating an underclass of medical labor. Postgraduate training posts were crucial for advanced training and experience for fellowship examination, not to mention for holding progressively responsible positions within the hospital service. While the proposed category permitted overseas doctors to practice medicine, their prospects of career development were uncertain. The board was concerned by the absence of any expectation or requirement of postgraduate training. The restrictions on the duration and type of posts to be held ran the risk of making overseas doctors "ineligible for rotational training schemes." This differential treatment advantaged domestic medical graduates in competition for training positions. Indeed, the stigma associated with a category of registration created for doctors with "inferior basic medical education" might circumscribe the career prospects of even those who pursued postgraduate training and quite possibly "prejudice any move towards making all junior hospital posts training posts." In short, the conditions of service associated with limited registration trapped overseas doctors into terminal junior posts, effectively creating a stratified career structure, one for British-trained and one for overseas-trained doctors.[47]

For its part, the Scottish Council regarded existing licensing or professional examinations as a far better instrument of assessment. Underlying its proposal was the assumption that success on a professional examination required a command of the English language. This model could also accommodate senior overseas doctors by modifying the content of the examination. Further, overseas doctors with a higher qualification, such as an M.R.C.P. or F.R.C.S., would be eligible for full registration provided that they satisfied the necessary clinical experience.[48] This Scottish Council response and other feedback did not bode well for moving forward on the special committee's new arrangements as a basis for amending legislation.[49] Cohen had planned to present the report to his council in November as a preliminary step to securing legislation in the current session of Parliament. By October these plans were indefinitely deferred. Between July and October, deepening tensions over the regulation of the profession between the GMC and the BMA not only overshadowed overseas registration, but also led to a political crisis within British medicine itself.

Interests and Function: The BMA and the Regulation of the Medical Profession, 1972–75

The adoption of the retention fee, which had been endorsed by the BMA council and later approved by Parliament in July 1969, highlighted a split between the BMA leadership and its membership. The need to put the GMC on a sound financial footing—without recourse to government support—was a sufficient rationale for securing the BMA's endorsement of the fee from the *BMJ* and the leadership of the association for the Medical Amendment Bill. The fee was to come into effect in spring 1970. But the fee inflamed dissatisfaction among the rank and file, already frustrated about the lag between compensation and the rising costs associated with the practice of medicine. Tensions had reached such a point that the BMA council was unable to meet a Privy Council deadline of January 15 to confirm the intention of the membership to pay the fee. Seeking to secure consent, the BMA council called a special representatives meeting on February 11.[50] The political stakes were high. Members who refused to pay risked being struck off the register and as such unable to remain a member of the BMA. Such doctors would be prohibited from working in the hospital service or in private practice. If enough were struck off, the potential for disrupting the delivery of health care to the public increased. The loss of fees would almost ensure governmental intervention to rescue the GMC and hence sacrifice its independence, an outcome that the GMC sought to avoid.

The BMA council put two recommendations before the membership to address the immediate financial crisis while laying the ground for enhancing the leverage of the association in the future. The first accepted the fee set at two pounds and the second called for the direct election of the majority of the membership on the GMC.[51] In the ensuing discussion, members proposed several amendments that were far more pointed. Payment of the fee was to be contingent on three conditions: the direct election of a majority of members of the GMC council, adequate representation of directly elected members on the executive and other key committees, and a joint BMA-GMC review of the functions of the GMC, subject to the approval of the association.[52] During a long meeting, BMA council chair Ronald Gilson pleaded with members to separate the fee from the composition and governance issues given the looming deadline. Any change in the composition of the GMC would trigger a lengthy process because it would require amending legislation. This was not simply a practical matter for Gibson; it was strategic. By paying the fee, the profession would be in a better position to lobby the incoming Conservative government on a host of issues such as medical education and reforming the NHS.[53] Rather than immediately heeding Gibson's advice, however, members adopted an even more adversarial position. The association was "to advise members of the profession to withhold payment" in the event that the "annual retention fee was imposed against the medical profession's wishes."[54] Before the meeting adjourned, a compromise amendment was finally proposed and adopted whereby the association agreed to approve the fee for the first year only.[55]

In linking the payment of the retention fee to conditions, the association was seeking to exercise leverage over the GMC. But this tactical maneuver created a standoff with the GMC. As president of the council, Cohen conceived of his role as defending a nongovernmental system of professional regulation while protecting the public. The retention fee was presented as a necessary means to retain its independence and carry out its functions. As the GMC continued to struggle financially, the passage of the Medical Act and activation of the fee reinforced Cohen's determination. The GMC prepared letters—dated February 1970—to medical professionals informing them of the fee, although holding them back until the Privy Council approved the implementation regulations. Under the provisions of the act, doctors had a window of fifty-six days to pay the fee. The council reserved the right to erase from the register those who failed to pay unless exempted.

The government sought a political solution, one that ensured the revenue from the fees and addressed the composition and governance of the GMC. On February 24, 1970, Crossman sounded out BMA council chair Gibson and president Derek Stevenson about a possible conference of principal representatives of British medicine including the BMA and the chief nonuniversity licensing bodies in Britain and Ireland.[56] After meeting with Cohen, Sir George Godber, the chief medical officer, felt that compromise seemed remote. Just as the association was dug in, Cohen did not appear to be in mood to compromise. He viewed the conference as a sign of the loss of ministerial confidence in his handling of the situation.[57]

Even as Cohen ultimately agreed to attend the conference, contingency plans were being developed. A representative of the ministry, P. Brenner, met with GMC registrar Martin Draper.[58] The conference was understood as a political gesture that acknowledged the views of the association while making the payment of the retention fee at least slightly more palatable. Neither Brenner nor Draper was confident that the conference would yield a solution to the satisfaction of all parties concerned. It was for this reason that both thought a public inquiry would provide a solution to the current standoff. Brenner doubted that an independent committee would endorse a directly elected council, as the purpose of the GMC was to protect the public, not advance the interest of the profession. This outcome would at least provide political cover for separating the condition from payment of the retention fee.[59]

The conference took place on March 11, 1970.[60] Godber presided on behalf of Crossman. The purpose of the meeting was explicit: "to make acceptance of the annual retention fee contingent on a change to the constitution of the GMC and its committees." Participants included representatives from the BMA, the GMC, the Royal Colleges, the Committee of Hospital Medical Staff, and the General Medical Staff Committee. As reported in a department summary, each was permitted time to present views on the matter from their institutional perspective. Predictably, the BMA and the GMC offered competing rationales. The BMA's Gibson stressed that the fee merely provided an occasion for what was described as a "widespread strong view that the GMC's role particularly in relation to other bodies, needed to be spelled out more definitely and the major part of its membership must be clearly seen to be elected by the profession."[61] Cohen contested that position and stated that, in fact, the purpose of the council was "to protect the public." In responding to the charge that the council was not responsive to the profession, he reminded the conference that as early as May 1969 he initiated a conversation and later embraced the principle of expanding the number of elected members from eleven to nineteen out of a total of forty-six members precisely because he "felt strongly about the importance of the part which such members should play in judging matters of serious professional misconduct." Still, Cohen opposed proposals that the majority of the council be elected directly. In his view, the voice of the profession was indirectly augmented by the college representatives that members freely elected. He pointed out that the age profile of existing elected members did not bode well for an expanding profession. They were, he noted, "significantly older than the rest of the GMC." Rather than making the council more representative, it would become less so at a time when the number of new members to the medical profession was growing. In closing, Cohen argued that the dispute over fees was a disruptive political gambit.[62]

Even though Cohen and Gibson approached the issue of expanding membership of the council from different points of view, representatives of other bodies concurred with the proposal of increasing the size of the council. Modifying the structure of the council permitted new or largely overlooked professional communities to be represented, according to Walpole Lewin, representing the Consultants Committee on Hospital Medical Staff. J. C. Cameron, who spoke on behalf of the General Medical Services Committee, hoped that change would lead to greater attention to the education and training of general practitioners while ensuring that their experience would be reflected in the disciplinary function of the council. As Brenner and Draper predicted, the conference did not yield an immediate solution, but it did build consensus for continuing to try. The representatives agreed to establish a working party to explore a new configuration of the council and, if necessary, the functions of the GMC. To underscore the seriousness of the undertaking, Godber sought an agreement from BMA president Stevenson for an independent inquiry in the event that the BMA membership rejected the working party recommendations.[63] This condition placed Stevenson in a difficult position. In light of the consensus reached at the conference, declining Godber's condition would have implied that the association was less interested in a solution for all of British medicine than in its narrow political interests. Conversely, accepting the condition meant that the association would be bound by the recommendations of the independent working party or those of public inquiry. Stevenson agreed.[64]

Led by Sir Brynmor Jones, vice chancellor of the University of Hull and a lay member of the GMC, the working party group included three representatives each from the BMA, universities, and colleges.[65] One year after the conference, in March 1971, the working party produced recommendations that addressed the demands of the association without altering the GMC's purpose. To this end, the party recommended expanding membership but rejected shifting from a mixed model of representation to wholly direct election: "The Working Party does not think it would be right for the Council to contain a majority of members directly elected by the profession who might in certain circumstances be tempted to regard their role as predominately one of protecting professional interests."[66] Instead, the recommendations that the working party forwarded to the secretary of state increased the total GMC membership from forty-seven to sixty-seven. This increase provided for twenty-nine directly elected members, or one more than the combined number for licensing bodies and universities. The report also recommended increasing the number of lay member appointments by the Crown from three to five, while the number of Crown-appointed medical members remained unchanged.[67] As for the representation of elected members on the key committees, the report accommodated the profession. On the twelve-member executive committee, they were to enjoy equal representation with the universities and colleges, or five members. In reference to the Finance Committee, which usually consisted of the president and treasurer of the council and a second treasurer for the branch councils in Scotland and Ireland, the report proposed that at least one of the two treasurers be a directly elected member. On the statutory committees as well, provision was made for the profession. On the Education Committee, the colleges (3) and universities (4) comprised the majority of seven, but five members were to be from the profession, whereas on the twenty-two member disciplinary committee, directly elected members would be in the majority with twelve. Even on the five-member penal cases committee, which included the president and one member of the profession, the report proposed replacing the three territorial representatives with membership by election.[68]

The momentum coming out of the work of the Brynmor Jones working party appeared to augur a compromise. Within months the GMC used its authority to implement some of the recommendations. These included increasing the number of elected members of the Education Committee to five and adding an elected member to the Finance Committee.[69] Meanwhile, in March 1972 the incoming Conservative secretary of state Keith Joseph indicated his willingness to seek amending legislation for expanding the number and the method of selection to the council.[70]

Differences that appeared to be patched up were reopened over the projected revenue shortfall and proposed fee increases. The two-pound retention fee that the association agreed to pay in 1970 was in fact not the preferred fee of the GMC. Cohen had originally set the fee at 3 pounds to ensure sufficient revenue to cover estimated expenditure for the council's statutory functions, general administration, and the effect of inflation. While 2 pounds was politically convenient, it proved to be ill-advised. The Joint Finance and Establishment Committee projected an accumulated deficit of 474,720 pounds for the period between 1971 and 1974. The difference between income and expenditure highlighted again the importance of overseas doctors to the operations of the GMC. In 1971 retention fees accounted for 110,000 pounds and 63,000 pounds for initial registration fees, while fees for all categories of registration for overseas doctors amounted to 113,500 pounds. The expenditure totaled 342,700 pounds with the following categories accounting for one-third of the total: general administration, statutory functions (discipline, education, and registering overseas doctors), and maintaining the register. These expenditures were expected to increase due to a variety of factors, including updating the register, administrating the retention fee, the costs associated with the presumed expansion of the council, and inflation.[71]

The GMC therefore proposed fee increases for registration and retention. The proposed fees were to increase 60 percent for all categories, or 10 pounds for initial registration, 15 pounds for full registration after completion of the provisional period, and 25 pounds for full registration. The retention fee was to be increased by 40 percent to 5 pounds—though the exemption for doctors during the provisional period remained unchanged—and a 30 percent fee increase for the restoration of names removed from the register for failure to pay. For overseas qualified doctors, the council proposed increases to the existing differential fees for initial registration: 40 percent for provisional registration, or 15 pounds, and 7 percent for full registration after the provisional period, or 20 pounds. Full registration fees increased 57 percent to 35 pounds. The fees associated with temporary registration were based on the length of the appointment: 5 pounds up to five months and 15 pounds for over twelve months. Another 2-pound fee was assessed for either renewal or extension of the temporary registration certificate for appointments lasting between five and twelve months. Of the three temporary registration fees, the council recommended reducing the fee for appointments up to twelve months to 10 pounds due to the disparate costs that such overseas doctors bore when changing positions. This reduction translated into a projected decrease of some 15,000 pounds in income.[72]

The proposed fee increases elicited frustration from the rank and file of the BMA and reinforced the call by the association for a review of the functions of the GMC. Since 1970 the association's position on fees was to pay "on a year to year basis without prejudice to the future." While this clause implied a measure of conditional agreement, the fees were legally binding as provided by the Medical Act. The GMC was quite open about its financial position, inviting the association's chief accountant to review its ledgers and statements. Even though the association's accountant concurred, this did not make the proposed increase in fees any more tolerable. If anything, it exacerbated suspicion that the GMC was poorly managed and that its functions were in need of an overhaul.[73] To this end, the BMA council not only requested that the Privy Council scrutinize the GMC's accounts but also began formalizing the ground for reviewing its functions through a working party led by association treasurer Solomon Wand. Wand's recommendation for a detailed review did not come as a complete surprise in light of the BMA membership's long-standing dissatisfaction with the GMC's oversight of registration, discipline, and education.[74]

The GMC was cooperative. Consideration of the functions of the GMC was part of the agreement that led to the Brynmor Jones working party. Cohen, too, was not unaware of Wand's working party. Gibson reported to the BMA council that Cohen had pledged to "give it every consideration. If there were ways of improving the functions of the Council within the present Act, he would consider them with BMA representatives."[75] While the leadership of the GMC and the association were continuing their cooperation, the association's representative body was far more restive.[76] Meeting in Southampton in July, BMA members considered the proposed annual retention fee as it had the past two years. But the timing of the increase provoked amendments from the floor deploring the proposed increase in fees before the review of GMC functions had been completed and proposing that the fee be replaced with public funding. The former amendment was carried; the latter failed. Before the meeting adjourned, a final resolution was adopted. It conditioned payment on the completion of yet another working party as well as a government inquiry into the regulation of the profession should the recommendations fail to be implemented in six months.[77]

This resolution was politically inflammatory. Up to this point, the association had not officially adopted a position to withhold paying the fee. Even though the fee was unpopular, it was paid for the most part. Some doctors engaged in a cat-and-mouse game with the GMC. But when the association was asked to assist in locating unresponsive doctors, it provided the addresses to the GMC.[78] At the same time, the GMC had not exercised its power to strike the names of delinquent doctors from the register. But the Southampton resolution escalated tensions between the association and the GMC. It not only challenged the authority of the GMC but also jeopardized its financial position. Politically, the appointment of a public inquiry into the regulation of the profession was a question of when, not if.

In the meantime, the working party led by Sir Ronald Tunbridge, chair of medicine at Leeds University and future association president, met and deliberated several times between July and November.[79] There is little evidence of the public tension between the organizations spilling over into the working party and its final report. Rather, the representatives of the GMC heard the suggestions of the association and clarified its position. This posture reflected the consensus about the statutory independence of the GMC and the fact that the association's suggestions either required ongoing discussions or amending legislation. This was the case in the matter of the registration of overseas doctors. Among the documents consulted was the February 1972 interim report of the special committee on overseas registration and the response of the BMA council. The working party acknowledged "problems" that would "require further discussion." Underlying these discussions was the assumption that the current system of overseas doctors' registration in general was flawed and that "future arrangements should no longer be based upon the concept of reciprocity." The position of the working group was clear about the next step. There was broad agreement in principle on the need for assessment, but further discussion was needed about means.[80] It is difficult to know whether this guarded optimism about resolving differences reflected compromise or its limits. But practically speaking, any substantive changes requiring fresh legislation had wide implications for British medicine. Echoing the March 1971 conference, the working party agreed that discussion about amending the Medical Act needed to be broadened to include not just representatives from the government but also other institutional interests implicated by the regulation of the profession, such as the university and nonuniversity licensing bodies and medical defense associations.[81]

The seeming compromise soon gave way to an impasse. Secretary of State Keith Joseph announced the appointment of a public inquiry into the regulation of the medical profession less than two weeks after the publication of the Tunbridge report. As Margaret Stacey has shown, the conflict over the retention fee prompted the government to bring forward amending legislation for revising the composition of the GMC while dooming future discussions about its functions.[82] In early November the GMC announced its intention to strike off dissident doctors who refused to pay their fees. The power was reserved to the council by virtue of the Medical Act, but the council had not theretofore exercised it. Up to the Southampton meeting, there had been no need. The association and the GMC had found a workable compromise to the retention fee: annual approval. The number of dissident doctors was not known, but one estimate put the number at four thousand or 7 percent of registered doctors. The decision to strike off doctors was not only within the rights of the GMC, but also conveyed a message of its determination to collect. Nor was the GMC opposed to a public inquiry. As early as 1970, it accepted an inquiry as an alternative way to resolve tensions about the composition of the council and its functions. Both the Brynmor Jones and the Tunbridge working parties endorsed the principle of an independent body charged with regulating the profession. A public inquiry was not without tactical advantages. It isolated dissident doctors who refused to pay the binding retention fee while at the same time constraining the association by broadening the discussion on the future of British medicine.

At least a month before Keith Joseph's announcement, the GMC had already reached the conclusion that amending legislation would not be forthcoming, particularly on overseas doctors' registration. The response to the February 1972 interim report raised doubts about the adoption of the recommendations, or even an uncontroversial bill in time before the end of the session of Parliament. As an alternative, the GMC decided to use its authority under the existing Medical Act to modify the conditions for overseas-trained doctors to secure temporary registration. Under this category of registration, the act empowered the GMC to use its discretion to determine the fitness of overseas-trained doctors from countries that did not reciprocate with Britain—that is, medical schools that were not subject to inspection by the GMC. In an October letter to Assistant Secretary of State for DHSS Robert Cattran, Draper outlined a variation of the GMC's arrangements for temporary registration as proposed in the interim report.[83] Elements of the nascent plan included a new examination to assess both the clinical and linguistic competence of overseas doctors together with an improved attachment period. Even as the committee of inquiry began its work, the GMC began exploring implementation with departmental personnel.

Conclusion

By the early 1960s, the context for the globalization of British medicine had shifted decisively. The openness to the world and in particular new Commonwealth countries that characterized the first decade and a half after the World War II was replaced by a widening preoccupation within and outside of the profession with policing the boundaries of domestic medicine. The system of overseas registration, the very instrument that transformed Britain into a Medical Mecca, came under increasing scrutiny and growing criticism. Some regarded the preferential treatment of overseas doctors from reciprocal Commonwealth countries as obsolete in the wake of decolonization. Still others portrayed the standards for temporary registration as unreliable. Even the Health Ministry, which relied on overseas doctors in the hospital service, was not immune to a discourse that openly questioned the competency of overseas doctors—regardless of the category of registration—to communicate in English and, by extension, practice medicine in the United Kingdom. Once regarded as representing British medicine as a world standard, overseas doctors were now portrayed as a threat to its professional integrity and patient safety. The 1965 adoption of the Clinical Attachment Scheme was designed to assure the public and the medical profession by having senior member of the medical staff supervise and assess the clinical and linguistic capacity of overseas doctors before they entered into their duties in the hospital service.

This shift, to be sure, reflected broad changes in Britain's global posture in the world and national identity at home. A set of policy choices redefined Britain's relationship with the Commonwealth. The Commonwealth Immigration Act of 1962 revised the unrestricted rights of citizens to travel and work in the United Kingdom for which the 1948 Nationality Act had provided. While doctors were treated preferentially under the voucher scheme to ensure a supply of labor for the hospital service, they—like other nonwhite residents of the Commonwealth—were subject to an animated discourse that called into question their capacity to be British. This was particularly the case in reference to their command of the English language. English competency served as a cultural commonsense litmus test that both enabled and entitled Britons—whether they were in the profession or not—to police membership within British nationality while reinforcing the status of nonwhite citizens as different.

The redefinition of the place of overseas doctors in British medicine was no less driven by the breakdown in consensus about the regulation of the profession by the GMC. Although the GMC was statutorily independent of the government, the conduct of its operations required the fee revenue of newly admitted doctors to the register. The fees deriving from the robust growth in the registration of overseas doctors supplemented those of domestic medical graduates whose overall numbers—and hence fees—had not changed very much from the prewar period. Until the early 1960s, the revenue from overseas registration masked the insecurity of the GMC. The drop in overseas fee revenue following the implementation of the 1962 Commonwealth Immigration Act exposed the hand-to-mouth existence of the GMC and spurred the development of a new revenue source, namely the annual retention fee. This fee, adopted in 1969, retained the names of doctors on the register, which legally entitled them to practice medicine.

In shifting the costs to all doctors on the register, who were overwhelmingly British-born and -trained, the GMC opened itself not only to criticism about its management, but also to calls from organized medicine to broaden its constitution and overhaul its functions. The association's insistence on making payment of the retention fee contingent on continuing conversations about institutional change aggravated political tensions between the association and the council. Ultimately, the failure to reach a compromise led to the appointment of a public inquiry into the regulation of the profession in 1971. Yet there was one area where the GMC, the BMA, and the government found compromise. This involved incorporating an assessment instrument into the registration process for overseas doctors. While the GMC had defended its administration of the register, by 1971 it initiated internal changes that were designed to treat overseas doctors differently. Lacking the power to repeal reciprocating relations with a sovereign country, the council instead used its existing authority over the category of temporary registration to impose an English language and clinical competency assessment test as a condition for admission for overseas doctors. Under growing scrutiny, the GMC—together with representatives of the nonuniversity licensing bodies—pressed ahead in developing and administering the Temporary Registration Assessment Board (TRAB) Test.

Chapter Seven

Redefining Access to the Medical Register for Overseas Medical Graduates, 1972–75

Introduction

For critics of the GMC, overseas doctors of color signified the collapse of the historical boundaries of nation and empire that had long restricted the practice of British medicine domestically to a distinct social group. Rather than expanding these boundaries in order to privilege white male doctors in the broader world, the register now facilitated the globalization of the profession within the domestic sphere. In aggregate, overseas doctors accounted for 51 percent of all admits to the full register between 1955 and 1966. Among member states in the Commonwealth, India and Pakistan were the leading exporting countries. In the medical and lay press, Indian and Pakistani doctors were unfavorably compared with doctors from nonreciprocating countries in Europe who practiced medicine under the far more restrictive terms of temporary registration. Their entitlement to full registration was deemed as little more than an obsolete privilege of a bygone imperial era when British doctors controlled the portals to Western medicine in colonial India. Decolonization not only yielded the modern nation-states of India and Pakistan but, it was feared, also diluted British medicine due to the purported national differences in medical education overseas.

Rendering these doctors into a globalized workforce suitable for Britain would involve dismantling their historically constructed access to the register as equals to domestic graduates. The retraction of reciprocity and the withdrawal of recognition would restrict medical graduates of India and Pakistan to the temporary register. Just as political imperatives informed the historical basis for opening the register to them, so too did the decision to narrow it. Even though calls for reforming the system of registration were framed in terms of buttressing the standards of medicine and ensuring patient safety, the GMC and policy makers were mindful of the internal contradictions of postwar British medicine: Britain's dependence on overseas medical labor in the face of growing demands from both the medical profession and the public to control that workforce. Although the respective decisions by the government to retract reciprocity from Pakistan in 1972 and by the GMC to withdraw recognition from Indian medical schools in 1975 were procedurally different, the net effect was the same: channeling access to the temporary register while keeping overseas medical labor under strict control in Britain. As I will show, the creation of the Temporary Registration Assessment Board (TRAB) test was crucial in reconstituting the boundaries of the register and recasting who was fit to practice British medicine.

Ending Reciprocity One Country at a Time: Pakistan, 1972

Changing domestic conceptions of Britishness paralleled and reinforced the political project of recasting the boundaries of British medicine. With the introduction of the 1962 Immigration Act, the role of race in determining membership within the British nation became more visible. To be sure, the voucher system provided officials with tools to check the flow of immigrants by adjusting the annual number of vouchers to be granted and by aligning preferred skills with countries of origin. The 1962 Immigration Act did not formally redefine the rights of Commonwealth citizens as provided for under the 1948 Nationality Act, which included the unrestricted right of permanent residence and the entry of dependents. As the decade unfolded, however, Labor and Conservative governments together with senior civil servants took steps that ultimately transformed nonwhite Commonwealth citizens into aliens by redefining membership within British nationality.

One of the earliest examples of this transformation was Britain's response to the forced migration of Kenyan nationals of European and South Asian descent from the east African country. The presence of both groups in Kenya was a product of British rule: Europeans who relocated served the colonial state and capitalized on generous access to farmland. South Asians, who migrated from British India, had formed an educated middle class and the backbone of a thriving commercial sector. In the wake of independence in 1963, the Kenyan government launched an Africanization campaign that spurred Kenyans of European and South Asian descent to flee in order to avoid discrimination. Technically, their British passports exempted them from the application of the 1962 Immigration Act. As such, they were entitled to unrestricted entry into the United Kingdom. Reflecting cabinet anxiety about the entry of South Asians into Britain, the government passed legislation in 1964 to protect the right of return of Kenyans of European descent. No such provision was made for Kenyans of South Asian descent. On the contrary, the Commonwealth Immigration Act of 1968 established a differential standard for nonwhite citizens of the Commonwealth. The right of return was reserved only for partials—that is citizens of the United Kingdom or Commonwealth with parents or grandparents who were born, adopted, or naturalized in the United Kingdom. This act, together with the Conservative government–sponsored Immigration Act of 1971, hollowed out the scope of the 1948 Nationality Act. As Kathleen Paul perceptively observed, "The act legally differentiated between the familial community of Britishness composed of the truly British—those descended from white colonizers—and the political community of British composed of individuals who became British through conquest or domination."[1]

For opponents of immigration, the departure of Pakistan from the Commonwealth in 1971 was more than a temporary breach within the voluntary association of member countries. It voided the very basis of British nationality that Pakistanis enjoyed in the United Kingdom. Pakistan's action—carried out in protest against British meddling in the Bangladesh war of independence—exposed the fundamentally unequal status of British Pakistanis as members of the British nation. Repatriation, according to one-time minister of health and relentless foe of immigration Enoch Powell, was a remedy for the "monstrous occurrence—the implanting in Britain without the assent or even knowledge of her people of a large growing Asian, West Indian and African population." While the government guaranteed the rights of Pakistani citizens already in the United Kingdom under separate legislation, the Immigration Act of 1971 still achieved its broader aim of narrowing access for Pakistanis seeking to enter Britain.[2]

Just as access to Britain became more conditional for nonwhite Commonwealth subjects, so too did access to British medicine. The Privy Council—based on the legal advice of the Foreign and Commonwealth Office—discontinued reciprocity with Pakistan on May 23, 1972.[3] Thereafter, medical graduates from Pakistan were ineligible for provisional or full registration. The only route left to them for entering the British medical market was through temporary registration. This applied to all Pakistani doctors—even those who were already in Britain awaiting registration.[4] Pakistan's withdrawal from the Commonwealth was a pretext, but not the cause, for the Privy Council's decision. Up to this time, reciprocity—as provided for in the 1896 Order in Council—withstood constitutional changes in the empire, not least of which was the creation of Pakistan and India as sovereign nation-states in 1947. The 1947 India Independence Act provided for the continuation of the order, subject to the agreement of participating countries. Even after Pakistan adopted the constitutional status as a republic in 1956—which ended the constitutional relationship between the British monarchy and the Pakistan state—there was no change. In fact, the application of part 3 of the Medical Act was not dependent on the constitutional status of countries. Allowance was made for countries that were within or outside the Commonwealth. As such, a country that seceded from the Commonwealth could continue to reciprocate under its existing order or a new order that reflected its status as a foreign country. This provision permitted South Africa, which withdrew from the Commonwealth in 1962 due to the opposition of member states to its apartheid regime, to resume reciprocating with Britain as a foreign country.[5]

The Privy Council had at least two courses of action available to it. Following the 1956 Act, it could allow the existing order to remain in force or replace it with a new one that recognized Pakistan as a foreign country.[6] Neither option was pursued because there was no political cost or pressing need. The prospect of a protest from the government of Pakistan on behalf of nationals in the United Kingdom was neither expected, given the strained bilateral relations, nor likely to have much of an impact domestically in light of the suspicion about the competency of overseas doctors. In any case, Pakistan was not a large source of overseas doctors for Britain.

Several months after the Privy Council's decision, interdepartmental tensions flared up over the legal basis of retraction. In October, lawyers from DHSS argued that Pakistan's membership status in the Commonwealth had no bearing on the application of part 3 of the Medical Act of 1956. Even though the NHS was far more reliant on India than Pakistan, the department was conscious of the negative impact of charges of discriminatory treatment against South Asian doctors, particularly in light of the effect of the 1962 Commonwealth Immigration Act. At an interdepartmental meeting, chaired by the clerk of the Privy Council, Sir Godfrey Agnew, the parties reached a consensus in the event that their differences could not be resolved. A new order restoring reciprocity would be produced while the dispute was forwarded to the Law Officers of the Crown for final disposition.

A new order was never produced.[7] Any new order would have required the GMC to recognize that foreign medical training met British qualifications for full or provisional registration.[8] Under mounting pressure, the GMC deployed its existing authority to scrutinize the medical schools of reciprocating countries, including Pakistan and India, to determine whether to continue recognizing their qualifications. At the same time, it spearheaded the development of an assessment test for admission to the temporary register for overseas medical graduates, including those from reciprocating countries whose qualifications the council had ceased to recognize. Collectively, these actions would redefine the relationship of overseas medical graduates to British medicine without having to officially terminate reciprocity.

Ending Reciprocity in All but Name: The GMC and the Redefinition of Fitness to Practice Medicine in the United Kingdom

Even though overseas doctors formed an important part of the activities and revenue of the GMC, until 1972 there was no dedicated committee oversight. The appointment of a special committee on overseas registration in the autumn of 1971 marked a new departure for the GMC. The committee was created in response to criticism about the presence of overseas doctors and, by extension, the alleged inadequacies of the GMC system of registration. The special committee's report sought to narrow the portal of entry into the medical market through a combination of internal changes and other adjustments that would require amending legislation by Parliament. The proposals included the creation of a dedicated standing committee on overseas registration. In February 1972, the council charged the new committee "to consider and determine on behalf of the Council all questions relating to the registration of doctors who qualified overseas."[9] When the council abolished the special committee later in November 1973, the overseas committee became the main policy-making body on overseas registration. In the meantime, the special committee report provided a template of the council's priorities.

One priority involved ascertaining the current standard of medical education at schools that had been previously approved for full or temporary registration.[10] Much of the institutional memory of the GMC was based on the inspection reports that had been undertaken at the request of schools when they sought recognition of their medical qualifications. By the time of the review, reciprocal arrangements existed among twenty-three countries, within and outside of the Commonwealth, which totaled seventy-eight medical schools.[11] Among the countries with reciprocity, India stood out with fifty-seven medical schools, or 73 percent of the total. Other countries with multiple schools included Australia, Canada, and Ceylon, with eight, four, and two respectively. The remaining six countries only had one school each. Little was known about these schools after the recognition of their qualifications.[12] During a two-decade period, just forty-three of seventy-three medical schools had been visited. In Canada, India, and South Africa, the council—respecting the autonomy of national licensing bodies—generally deferred to the judgment of national medical councils. Their approval was sufficient.[13] To address concerns about the deficiency of medical education in reciprocating countries, the committee decided to solicit further information from overseas medical schools.[14] Although the committee did not discuss the potential consequence for schools that failed to satisfy the equivalency expectation, the withdrawal of recognition of overseas qualifications for any form of registration—provisional or full registration—was a likely result.

While the overseas committee solicited information, Cohen focused attention on modifying the conditions of temporary registration. This topic was of particular concern to the special committee on overseas registration, not to mention a persistent target of criticism within the profession. The Medical Act gave the council the power to recognize overseas medical qualifications for the purpose of temporary registration. In the opinion of critics, the council was failing in its responsibility to protect the public. This criticism gave rise to calls for a less subjective and more objective assessment of overseas doctors along the lines of the United States Educational Council Foreign Medical Graduates (ECFMG) examination. Launched in 1956, the United States established this examination to regulate the access of foreign medical graduates to the United States. The examination assessed knowledge of medicine and English-language competency. What critics of the UK system of registration liked about the ECFMG examination was that applicants sat for the examination outside of the United States and passage on the exam was a condition for entry.

Although Cohen had rejected the US examination model, the GMC nonetheless embraced an assessment instrument for admissions to the temporary register.[15] An assessment test provided a politically acceptable tool for narrowing access to the medical market without breaching the terms of reciprocity. Under reciprocity, Britain could not impose a test on overseas-trained doctors from reciprocating countries as a condition of registration without jeopardizing the rights of British medical graduates in affected countries. Yet the council—as did equivalent authorities in reciprocating overseas countries—had the right to withdraw recognition from medical schools if the medical education failed to satisfy the standards of a British equivalent. In such cases, medical graduates from affected countries would be subject to any conditions, including passing an assessment test, as determined by the council for temporary registration. In short, the GMC could address the criticism of its oversight of overseas registration without formally abolishing reciprocity and potentially provoking an adverse response from India—Britain's chief exporting country for doctors. In a letter to Assistant Secretary Cattran, GMC registrar Draper connected the review to this outcome in India. "Before proceeding to withdraw recognition from these qualifications it would no doubt be requisite for the Council to attempt to satisfy themselves as to the standard of qualifications in question though it is thought unlikely that the authorities in India would be prepared to afford the necessary facilities, and even if visits were permitted the reports thereafter might not be favorable."[16]

For its part, the DHSS was well aware of the allegations about the clinical and linguistic competency of overseas-trained doctors. Addressing the problem of overseas doctors was as much in these doctors' interest as it was in the interest of the GMC: they staffed the hospital service and delivered preventive and curative medicine in general practice settings. It should therefore not come as a surprise that DHSS officials were open to language testing. Neither the department nor employing authorities were qualified nor formally tasked with this responsibility. Shifting language assessment to the GMC would minimize the department's responsibility for the competency of overseas doctors and, by extension, public criticism. It would also simplify the workload of employers and hospital authorities. Enforcement would now be linked to the "near-water tight registration procedures" that in turn would make clinical attachment redundant and likely to be abolished in the future.[17]

A format that weeded out doctors with English difficulties without discouraging qualified doctors seeking employment in Britain was optimal. P. Brenner suggested an initial informal evaluation in the sending country before formal testing in Britain. Such an evaluation had the advantage of establishing a common standard for all overseas doctors who sought either employment in the hospital service or in general practice.[18] Brenner intimated that Draper was open to the "idea of a simple form of language testing for doctors who have not been through clinical attachment and whose ability to speak English is prima facie suspected. Indeed, he is disposed to favor such arrangements, which he does not think should be too difficult to take."[19] Nor did the Foreign and Commonwealth Office see any insurmountable problems, according to Robertson: "The practical problem would be in mounting this examination in countries where the British Council do not have offices. If made formal, governments would suspect of us recruitment; educated people in the Middle East and the Indian sub-Continent all pride themselves on their English, and could resent being subjected to a formal test."[20]

Even as English-language assessment was a welcome development, ensuring the regular flow of doctors remained a high priority for the department. Cattran was worried that the GMC would reject out of hand any applicant who received a borderline initial evaluation. For this reason, he modified the evaluation format in ways that would accommodate the priorities of the department and the GMC. This involved placing the burden on doctors overseas to assume the risk to travel to Britain to sit for the examination while leaving it to the council to determine who, if anyone, would be exempted. The informal evaluation would not determine eligibility for the examination in Britain or exemption. Instead, it would afford prospective applicants for registration and the GMC with an additional source of information about their prospects of success.[21] Depending on the results of the informal evaluation, the GMC might exempt candidates from the formal examination.

Cattran was clear-eyed about the political symbolism of the proposals contemplated by the GMC: "All of these recommendations point the same way; to tightening up of the standards applied to overseas doctors wanting to practice in this country. Do not think there is much doubt that this would be broadly welcome to the profession, and probably, in itself, popular with the public." At the same time, the recommendations placed at risk the supply of overseas doctors and the delivery of health care: "But if in one way or another it excluded so many doctors who would otherwise have come here as to make it difficult to staff developments in the NHS or even force closures of services, that would not be so popular. There is therefore to some extent a 'quality versus quantity' element in which we will need to pay special attention to the quantity aspects because no-one else will, at least unless and until closures start."[22] Moreover, the consequences of withdrawing reciprocity were potentially more far-reaching, partly because of the importance of India as a source of overseas doctors and partly because recognition was strictly a matter for the GMC. Until the scope of withdrawal of recognition from medical schools in India was known, Cattran thought it best "to listen and to question a good deal before deciding what our definitive reaction must be."[23]

Underlying this wait and see approach was the recently initiated public inquiry on the regulation of the medical profession (known as the Merrison Commission after its chairman, Sir Alec Merrison), which was appointed in April 1973. As the chief regulatory body, the GMC would be placed under a public microscope focused on its governance and functions, including the registration of overseas doctors. When the committee would complete its work and report and whether the government would take up its final recommendations for amending legislation were questions yet to be answered. Meanwhile the GMC proceeded to weigh methods for scrutinizing overseas-trained doctors, including the exploration of individual testing for English-language and clinical competency. Testing not only marked a new departure, but also required consensus and cooperation among members of the GMC and other interested entities on a host of matters ranging from the type of test and component elements of the test to logistics. "All are agreed," according to Robertson's summary of his meeting with Draper, "there should be language testing and that this should not be a function of failing to consultant assessors [during the attachment period]. Beyond that, there seems to be no general view on control of professional skills. Some think that it would be sufficient to tighten up the attachment scheme; others want to be more radical and set up formal tests, based on multiple choice questionnaires, practical assessment and language testing." At the same time, Draper rebuffed any departmental effort to shape the process or prescribe its outcome. Declining Robertson's offer to have the department formulate a draft proposal, he preferred "to leave it to the colleges and other professional bodies to devise machinery for educational tests."[24]

The GMC and the Construction of the TRAB Examination

In February 1973, Cohen approached the examining boards of the principal professional colleges in England and Scotland—the Conjoint Examining Board in England, the Society of Apothecaries, and the Scottish Triple Board—to ascertain their interest in individual assessment of overseas-trained doctors. Unlike universities, these bodies neither granted degrees nor conducted basic biomedical research. They were instead professional bodies that administered membership examinations in medicine, midwifery, surgery, and apothecary for prospective new entrants as well as higher diplomas. These credentials conferred the stamp of approval of the professional colleges and by extension the wider medical profession as to professional competency. Their endorsement and participation in the operation of any testing regime was therefore crucial politically and practically.

In March, June, and July 1973, these representatives, along with others from the GMC and observers from the DHSS and the BMA, met to discuss the scope, nature, and logistics of assessing overseas doctors. These meetings yielded agreement in principle and a broad set of recommendations on testing. The assessment instrument was restricted to overseas doctors seeking temporary registration. It was to be conducted in English and designed to ascertain command of the English language for purposes of the practice of medicine in a clinical setting, and it would be administered ten times annually—every month except August and September—to a maximum of 150 candidates, for a total of 1,500 test takers per year. Separately, an improved clinical attachment scheme would continue to be administered by the DHSS and remain a condition of employment in the NHS hospital service unless exempted.[25]

The process of reaching consensus revealed different perspectives about nearly every aspect of assessment. Some felt that the proposed test did not go far enough in evaluating overseas doctors. Royal College of Surgeons Dean of the Faculty Cyril Scurr, who represented the Examining Board in England, insisted that all overseas doctors should be tested—not just those seeking temporary registration, but also those with recognized degrees from reciprocating countries. He raised the suggestion that the GMC consider withdrawing recognition from overseas medical schools. Vice Chancellor of London University and radiologist Brian Windeyer—who represented the Society of Apothecaries—added that in his opinion many overseas schools were simply unsatisfactory. Cohen reminded the committee that the GMC had no legal authority to require tests for all incoming doctors beyond those seeking temporary registration, but at the same time assured committee members that the overseas committee was scrutinizing information from medical schools in countries that enjoyed reciprocity.[26]

The discussion about the nature and structure of the test highlighted different priorities as well. What did fitness to practice mean and what was the best means to determine it? John Fry, a prominent member of the Royal College of General Practitioners, stressed the importance of an instrument that tested the ability of the candidate to work in the social setting of the hospital rather than strictly clinical competence or the ability to practice medicine. Could the candidate communicate with patients and family members, give directions to nurses and auxiliary personnel, and confer with other members of the medical staff? MacLean, who represented the Scottish Board of Management of the Scottish Triple Qualification, preferred a test modeled on the USFMG examination together with a separate patient-based clinical assessment.[27] The discussion about clinical competency also yielded a range of opinions about the best assessment format. Some thought the candidate's ability to make routine diagnoses was far more important than an ability to diagnose difficult cases. Others doubted that a supply of patients for the clinical demonstration portion of the assessment would be readily available. In the end, the majority opinion dropped patient-based clinical assessment as an integral part of testing. Thomas Hunt, chair of the English Board, found clinical assessment was "neither feasible nor essential." In a summary statement that acknowledged the racial preferences of patients, he noted that there was concern about "subjecting medical graduates to tests including the examination of patients, that there would in any case be some patient resistance, and that there would be a lack of uniformity in conducting such tests."[28]

No representative was willing to assume responsibility for the management of the test itself. Neither the medical colleges nor the GMC were prepared to assume financial responsibility. Draper closed off any discussion of using temporary registration fees as a subsidy. He was, however, willing to offer the staff and facilities of the GMC to process applications. As an alternative source of support, Draper floated the idea of approaching the DHSS. If testing proved to be successful, the savings from ending the clinical attachment scheme might in whole or partly be redirected to the test. In the meantime, all agreed on self-funding through testing application fees. While a fee of 25 or 30 pounds was suggested, setting the precise amount was deferred until more information about the estimated costs of the test could be collected, and it would then be determined whether the administration was to be based strictly on operating costs or generating a slight surplus. These details were delegated to two sub-committees: one on testing administration and one on the elements of the test itself.

Separately, representatives of the Royal Colleges and Society of Apothecaries met to consider the proposed test. For the most part, their March 1974 report clarified the features of the examination and the structure of assessment that had been agreed upon, including the supplemental role of an improved clinical attachment scheme. The examination, provisionally designated Temporary Registration Assessment, consisted of four parts:

Part I: Comprehension of spoken English (1/2 hour)
Part II: Factual professional knowledge (1 1/2 hours)
Part III: Ability to understand written English and to write it intelligibly (1 hour)
Part IV: A viva voca examination of practical, rather than factual, professional knowledge (20 minutes).[29]

Apart from the test of linguistic competency, the licensing bodies were to appoint a panel of assessors tasked with assessing the medical knowledge of each candidate. Safeguards to ensure consistent standards included the circulation of examiners among different testing venues in the United Kingdom and the confidential nature of candidate reports. The reports would form part of the dossier that the council would evaluate when making its decision on registration. The separation of assessment from the registration decision was designed to introduce greater objectivity or, at least to minimize subjectivity, in the decision making of the GMC.

As for the administration of testing, the working group proposed the establishment of a Temporary Registration Assessment Board (TRAB). Logistical as well as financial concerns spurred this recommendation. The group endorsed an independently funded board with narrowly defined responsibility, believing it would be better suited to expedite the development and implementation of the testing regime. The board would allow for members or advisors whose expertise would be critical to the operation of the test, including the Royal Colleges of Obstetrics and Gynecology, the University of London Institute of Education, and representatives of the British Postgraduate Medical Federation and other bodies as needed. At the same time, the group made it quite clear that the proposed board would not supplant the registration authority of the GMC or impose any financial or administrative responsibilities on the colleges themselves. They were to do "no more than to conduct a T.R. Assessment and to report its findings confidentially to the G.M.C. with its recommendations."[30]

The DHSS was broadly pleased with the outline of the TRAB. The board provided a unified management structure. Quite apart from avoiding additional workload and personnel costs to the department, the board would manage the examination process in all facets, ranging from coordinating the monthly examinations and the assignment of examiners to scheduling candidates and granting exemptions.[31] Ideally, candidates would sit and pass the test before entering into an attachment for four weeks at a designated hospital. This sequence saved time and money by reserving slots for those who were likely to be granted registration rather than for those who failed. Still, the department had concerns about the coordination of the test with the clinical attachment scheme.

The department faced a chronic backlog of applicants for attachment. Its clearing house processed applications on a first come, first served basis unless there was a specific request from a hospital employing authority. But the maximum number of attachments was 1,500 a year. In hopes of working through the backlog, the department in May 1972 deferred accepting new applications for six months. At the end of this period, the deferral was made indefinite. The list was reduced by 1,000 or more applications, but this was not a reliable solution. Britain ran the risk of discouraging new applicants without being certain whether any of the 14,000 on the attachment waiting list remained interested.[32]

Recent totals for temporary registration applicants and attachments were well above the projected 1,500 maximum number of test takers and attachment slots annually available. In 1973 the GMC granted some 2,250 temporary registration certificates. Of the 7,331 applications for attachment, 1,535 were completed and another 2,067 were exempted.[33] Given the labor needs of hospitals and the demand for attachments, bringing the number of test takers into parity with attachment slots would require a generous use of exemptions.[34] But such exemptions fed into criticism about the lax oversight of the register and the appointment of doctors to the hospitals service. There was also concern that the wait time between sitting for the test and the announcement of results would stall the movement of doctors to their attachment assignments while imposing a financial burden on candidates for registration. The wait might discourage not only those who passed but also others from traveling to Britain for employment in the NHS. Either scenario would reinforce the frustrations of employing authorities and consultants who complained about overseas doctors not showing up for or completing their attachment period.[35]

The Home Office raised related concerns. Under existing work permit rules, twelve- month and six-month stays were available to overseas doctors with either a previous arrangement position or a confirmed attachment slot. Extensions were possible for both categories. At a meeting with department officials, Prosser raised concerns about doctors who failed the test. They could not only remain in the country for a prolonged period under the work permit rules but were also entitled to request an extension of their stay. Even the refusal of an extension did not necessarily mean their immediate removal due to their right of appeal, which could take several additional months. There was also the risk that these doctors might seek employment either in the health service or in another sector of the economy. Whether they pursued this course or not, their presence would still be an embarrassment and costly to the DHSS, which would be required to provide a supplementary benefit to them during the appeal process.[36]

Talks between representatives from the GMC and the DHSS produced a compromise, one that served their respective priorities: restoring the credibility of the GMC oversight of the register and addressing staffing needs of the hospital service.[37] All overseas doctors seeking temporary registration were required to sit for the test unless exempted by the GMC. But the department secured an important concession at a moment when the withdrawal of recognition from India was a foregone conclusion. All candidates for the TRAB test had to have a prearranged attachment place. This prerequisite enabled the department to make use of its extensive attachment waiting list in order to minimize the interruption in the supply of doctors for the service. A sample analysis of the fourteen thousand applicants for clinical attachment revealed that ten thousand were likely to be eligible for full registration. Under the existing GMC policy, these doctors would be exempted from the TRAB test because they possessed a recognized qualification for full registration from a reciprocating country. As Joan Firth has noted, these doctors would in turn provide a "reserve of fully registrable doctors to feed into the attachment places."[38]

Still, the DHSS had to walk a fine line between openly recruiting overseas doctors and portraying the opportunity costs associated with seeking employment in the United Kingdom. It subtly managed this feat. When informing doctors on the waiting list about the new conditions for temporary registration or the need to contact the GMC to apply, the department conveyed the relative advantages of full registration for those who were eligible. The fifty-pound test fee was in addition to the registration fees. Prospective candidates were also strongly advised of the need to "have sufficient money to cover the cost of the test, the cost of accommodation in this country while awaiting an attachment place and the cost of their return fare home if they fail to complete the test or attachment satisfactorily." The message was clear: full registration exempted doctors from the TRAB test and expedited employment opportunities in the hospital service.[39]

For its part, the GMC would determine test exemptions based on the applicant's qualifications and experience. It was only after this stage that regional hospital authorities would be offered the names of applicants to recruit for attachments. They would, in turn, schedule their test. Sensitive to the time constraints of employing hospital authorities and candidates alike, the department recommended that test scheduling be as practically close as possible to their arrival time in the United Kingdom. Although the preferred sequence was for candidates to sit for the test and then enter into the attachment period while waiting for test results, the department acknowledged that this sequence would be under ideal circumstances. During the attachment period, authorities were urged to encourage candidates to make "provisional arrangements for their first hospital post in sufficient time for them to vacate the accommodation as soon as attachment is completed."[40]

While the attachment prerequisite insulated the DHSS from wild swings in the availability of doctors, the department still faced a credibility problem with the attachment scheme. Seeking cooperation with Joint Consultants Committee (JCC), it intended to improve the scheme by making it a more rigorous assessment experience. But the JCC refused to cooperate, deeming attachment "an ineffective means of ensuring the adequacy of overseas doctors."[41] This view was by no means one that could be ignored. With a membership consisting of nominees from the English and Scottish Royal Colleges along with Royal College of Obstetricians and Gynaecologists and the British Dental Association, the JCC comprised the institutional leadership of the elite of the British medical profession. The committee operated as the chief conduit of communication between the Ministry of Health and hospital staff and negotiated a wide range of medical and organizational subjects. Given the role of senior staff and consultants in the attachment scheme, their endorsement was essential. If anything, their criticism of the scheme enhanced their leverage with the department. Attachment critics regarded the exemption categories as too broad and the failure rate too low. The personal connection forged between the attached doctor and a single assessor compromised objectivity and precluded standardized norms of competency. Nor was the remuneration of senior staff assessors regarded as commensurate with their degree of labor and responsibility.

The department was well aware of these criticisms. Cattran embraced the TRAB test in part because it provided a practical long-term replacement of the attachment scheme and its attendant headaches. The decision by TRAB to omit a clinical component effectively meant that the scheme would have to be improved. Lacking the requisite competency, the department deferred to the GMC. The changes proposed by Draper included the addition of a second consultant assessor, standardization of the assessor reports, and the regular incorporation of these reports in the deliberations for granting temporary registration for first time or its renewal for continuing doctors.[42]

For the GMC, the JCC vote of no confidence in the existing attachment scheme added a complication but did not doom the TRAB test. TRAB was tailored to address a problem, namely assessing the competency of overseas doctors to practice medicine in a hospital setting as part of the temporary registration process. Broad agreement existed about the need for individual assessment, and representatives from the chief licensing bodies had developed a test for this purpose. The position of the council remained unchanged even as Sir John Richardson succeeded Lord Cohen as president. The crucial question for the GMC was not so much if but when the test could be administered.

At the request of the DHSS, Draper in October forwarded a revised attachment scheme to the JCC for consideration. While the JCC considered the proposal, it agreed to suspend its decision to withdraw support from the attachment scheme. Yet in the ensuing months of planning for coordinating attachment as a prerequisite for the TRAB test, DHSS officials could not guarantee that the changes to attachment would be in place in time for the June test.

From this point, the GMC unilaterally decided on decoupling the attachment requisite. At the open meeting of the council on November 14, Richardson confirmed publicly for the first time a testing administration scheduled for the coming June. While department officials were aware of this timing, they were caught completely off guard by the report that the council had decided that the prearranged attachment would no longer be a prerequisite for the test.[43] This decision certainly reflected the delay due to the JCC's reluctance to participate. It was also a political tactic to remove any remaining doubts about proceeding with the TRAB test.

When the JCC took up the proposed revised attachment scheme in January, TRAB was separated from attachment. As an invited guest, Richardson stressed the need to improve the safeguards for the public as proposed in the revised scheme. Building on a consensus that overseas doctors who sought posts in hospital services needed to be assessed, he argued that the revised scheme provided a corrective to the earlier version's acknowledged deficiencies. The implication of the position of the JCC was made clear. Opposition placed public safety in peril. Should consultants refuse to participate, their oversight of the competency of overseas doctors would revert to the era before the adoption of clinical attachment in 1966: "If there were no possible time [to improve the scheme] the G.M.C. thought that the present scheme better than nothing."[44]

Richardson's appeal yielded mixed results. The committee still refused to see attachment as sufficient and insisted on the addition of a clinical component to TRAB. However, the JCC did agree to consult with the GMC to explore possible interim arrangements.[45] Under the interim arrangements the JCC proposed, the TRAB score would determine the nature of attachment and whether a second full TRAB examination would be necessary. For those whose score was above the 75 percentile, attachment would serve as an orientation to the NHS. Those whose score was within the 25 percentile would not proceed further and "should not remain in the United Kingdom." Candidates with scores between 25 percent and 75 percent would complete a full attachment. Their progress toward registration, however, depended on the assessor's report and whether their original scores were high enough to warrant a second sitting of the TRAB. Only those with high enough scores would proceed further.[46]

While considering the JCC proposal, Richardson and Hunt met with the Comitia of the Royal Colleges of Physicians.[47] Politically, the support of the Comitia was important insofar as the college was represented on the JCC and on the TRAB. It would buttress the course of action undertaken by the GMC. As chair of the TRAB, Hunt reminded the fellows that the test was the product of the consensus of the working group from the five professional colleges that comprised the examining bodies. To date, the board had made considerable progress in nominating assessors for the examination centers in Edinburgh, London, and Manchester while actively supporting strengthened assessment for doctors seeking appointments in the service. He insisted that attachment was a more manageable and effective method "of assessing a candidate's practical clinical proficiency than a ten minute examination in Queen's Square over a rather artificial out-patient set-up."[48] As Richardson implied in his remarks to the JCC, Hunt added that the position of consultants ran the risk of exposing the public to even more poorly trained or qualified overseas doctors. In the report of his remarks, he "hoped that the Comitia might feel that the proposals were a great deal better than the present situation, they might indeed not be perfect but they would gradually modify and adapt as time went on." For his part, Richardson did not want to create a confrontation between the Comitia and the JCC, but rather to improve conditions for negotiating with it. He appealed to the Comitia to refrain from public comment that would complicate his efforts to persuade the JCC that the examination "conducted by the three great non-university examining bodies of this country with all the expertise that they and they alone in non-University circles had, was better than nothing."[49]

Their remarks elicited extensive commentary from fellows. For the most part, the comments reiterated the inadequacy of oversight for overseas doctors at the point of registration and in the service. Dr. Emerson noted that the underlying problem with attachment for the JCC was the lack of quality control, noting the low failure rate and potential for the assessor to develop personal ties with the attached doctor.[50] Stressing public safety, former college president Sir Selwyn-Clarke urged the adoption of a revised attachment for overseas doctors before "they were released on the public and it was the duty of the consultants to get these schemes going."[51]

There were other indicators that the existing registration system insufficiently enforced standards. The uneven performance of overseas doctors on the Conjoint examination troubled J. L. M. Riordan. Sixty-six percent of overseas doctors did not pass compared to 13 percent of British graduates.[52] To underscore the need for greater quality control in evaluating all overseas doctors, Riordan pointed out that the failure rate for fully registered doctors was similar to those who were temporarily registered. Echoing Riordan, Dr. Thould insisted that the TRAB set a high standard to distinguish licensed overseas doctors from other candidates and to ensure their credibility when working alongside British graduates.[53]

The lack of confidence in the training of overseas doctors together with the narrow focus of TRAB on doctors seeking temporary registration justified the use of other ways to control access to practice in the United Kingdom. Richardson did not disagree with the need to examine doctors who were entitled to full registration, but the Medical Act limited what the

GMC could do. He noted that the council also called for amending the Medical Act. In the meantime, Richardson intimated the willingness of the council to withdraw recognition from overseas medical schools—even those from reciprocating countries—that failed to meet its standards of medical education.[54] Richardson felt confident that this proposed outline for legislation, if endorsed by the Merrison Committee and provided for by Parliament, would more than meet the concerns of the JCC about safeguarding access to the register.[55] By the end of the meeting, Richardson and Hunt left with the support of the Comitia.

Shortly after meeting with the Comitia, Draper informed JCC deputy secretary Gullick that Richardson intended to forward his proposal to the full council for consideration. In the meantime, he noted that Richardson estimated that at least six months would be needed to plan and operate the JCC model even if it were deemed to be feasible. Even though Richardson knew that Gullick regarded TRAB as incomplete without some form of clinical assessment, he was confident that the TRAB would proceed as planned.[56] In notifying Joan Firth, Draper wrote that "in these circumstances, and because the present clinical attachment scheme is becoming increasingly unable to provide a reliable screening procedure, the Committee concluded that it was imperative that the tests being devised by the TRAB should be brought into operation as soon as possible."[57] Given the department's deference to and dependence on the GMC, this rationale seemed little more than a weak justification for subordinating the department's need to the GMC's when it became convenient. In a memo to a departmental colleague, Firth acidly noted, "I do not propose to rise to the bait that 'the present clinical attachment scheme is becoming increasingly unable to provide a reliable screening procedure.'" She added that "the GMC have taken their decision; it will be interesting to see whether they implement it."[58]

Conclusion

The TRAB test represented a reassertion of the authority of the GMC to regulate access to the domestic medical market. Its development took place in a policy-making environment that had become much more amenable than ever before to redefine membership in British society and medicine. A succession of immigration legislation transformed Commonwealth citizens into aliens who possessed few of the rights provided for in the comparatively open 1948 Nationality Act. This change, which was sponsored by both Labor and Conservative governments, underscored the growing hostility to a multiracial population in the United Kingdom. Instead of redefining British nationality as multiracial, policy makers erected barriers to the entry and settlement of nonwhite Commonwealth citizens, including South Asians and West Indians.

The boundaries of British medicine were redefined at the same time. Reference to the language competency of overseas doctors, especially those from India and Pakistan, long functioned as a surrogate for race, one that tacitly highlighted the differences between overseas doctors and domestic medical graduates. This discourse reinforced the fiction of the homogeneity of British medicine and the threat posed by the heterogeneity of overseas doctors to the British public. Questions about language competency in clinical settings not only raised doubts about patient safety but also validated concerns about the suitability of medical education afforded in major reciprocating countries. By the end of the 1960s, there was broad consensus among the medical establishment, organized medicine, and senior governmental officials about the need to scrutinize the credentials of overseas medical graduates to verify their competency to practice medicine in the United Kingdom.

Translating this consensus into effect was contingent on several entities whose authority and interests were not necessarily identical. The Privy Council determined whether Britain reciprocated with other countries. The GMC, in turn, was empowered to recognize the qualifications for admission to the provisional or full register. Dependent on the labor of overseas doctors, the DHSS in 1969 mandated the completion of a clinical attachment as a condition of appointment in the hospital service. Senior hospital-based consultants assessed the attached overseas doctors, using their professional credibility to legitimate the competency of overseas doctors to practice medicine. This distribution of responsibilities produced tensions over the best means to police the boundaries of British medicine. In retracting reciprocity from Pakistan in 1971, the Privy Council retaliated against Pakistan's decision to withdraw from the Commonwealth. It was a convenient opportunity to narrow access to the medical market in a domestic climate that had grown increasingly hostile to nonwhite doctors. For its part, the DHSS objected to the Privy Council's decision. A consensus was reached that conditioned any final decision about restoring reciprocity with Pakistan on the assessment of the GMC. The GMC declined to extend recognition.

This decision was hardly a surprise. The GMC pursued a strategy to bring overseas medical graduates, especially from India, more directly under its control. To this end, its newly created overseas registration committee reviewed the medical education in twenty-three reciprocating countries. Failure to meet standards that would satisfy the GMC provided a pretext for achieving the same outcome as retracting reciprocity but without the potential political fallout that the DHSS feared. Stripped of the automatic right to provisional or full registration, overseas doctors would have to pass a TRAB test, an instrument designed to assess their fitness to practice medicine in the United Kingdom. The test also ensured an elastic pool of medical labor to meet the staffing needs of the hospital service of the NHS. As the next chapter will show, the withdrawal of GMC recognition from Indian medical school removed the last hurdle to completely redrawing the boundaries of British medicine.

Chapter Eight

Managing a Globalized Workforce within the National Boundaries of British Medicine, 1975

Introduction

The GMC proceeded with redefining how overseas-trained doctors gained access to the register at a moment of political crisis within British medicine. On November 23, 1972, Secretary of State for Health and Social Security Sir Keith Joseph announced in Parliament the appointment of a committee of inquiry into the regulation of the medical profession. The committee, chaired by Sir Alec Merrison, was created to follow up on a pledge by Joseph's predecessor, Richard Crossman, in March 1969, during the continuing dispute between the BMA and the GMC over the retention fee. Crossman had urged the association leadership to find common ground with Lord Cohen to resolve differences over the governance structure and functions of the GMC. Working groups had reached consensus on a host of items—including the centrality of an independent body to regulate the medical profession—prior to Secretary Joseph's announcement. But the hardening of opposition to the fee among a core element within the BMA membership, together with the intention of the GMC to remove nonpayers from the register, effectively doomed compromise. The specter of an apparent breakdown in the regulation of the profession was not without liabilities for the government. While the number of doctors to be potentially removed was not definitively known, even the possibility carried the threat of a contraction in the supply of registered doctors and a possible interruption in the delivery of health care to the public. At a minimum, the appointment of the Merrison Committee was a means to defuse a crisis while grounding any proposed changes to the regulation of the profession in the judgment of a nonpartisan body that represented a cross section of the public and the profession, but neither the GMC nor BMA.

The inquiry was unprecedented in the longer than 150–year history of the GMC. Although the GMC would be subject to prolonged scrutiny, council president Lord Cohen and his successor, Sir Richardson, welcomed the inquiry. This was not simply a matter of putting on a brave face in a difficult situation. However much the GMC and the BMA were at odds about governance and oversight functions, there was broad agreement on at least two principles. First, the regulation of the medical profession should remain the responsibility of an independent body. The second concerned admission to the register. All overseas-trained doctors, it was agreed, should be subjected to more scrutiny, including testing, before being admitted to the register. Still, there were unknowns about the outcome of the public inquiry. What recommendations the committee would propose and whether the government in power would introduce any new amending legislation would ultimately be subject to the vagaries of parliamentary politics. The piecemeal nature of previous amending legislation did not augur for swift action.

As I will discuss, this uncertainty created a political space for the council to seize the initiative. Rather than tabling the recommendations of the overseas committee, the council expedited their implementation. After a review of the medical qualifications awarded in twenty-three countries in the Commonwealth, the committee in May 1975 recommended withdrawing GMC recognition from the fifty-two medical schools in India due to the unresponsiveness of the Medical Council of India to the requests from the GMC for information. The council's eventual adoption of this recommendation meant that any Indian graduates seeking access to the medical market would be required to pass the TRAB examination and be bound to the conditions associated with employment in the NHS—namely, the completion of a clinical attachment as well as restrictions on the duration and scope of appointment.

By 1972 Commonwealth doctors in general and Indian doctors in particular were increasingly seen as a globalized labor force—a temporary adjunct to the British medical profession. Immigration legislation not only rolled backed their rights to work and settlement but also redefined their perceived relationship within the community of British nationals. Nor could they look to their home government to shield them against any arbitrary decision that circumscribed their right to practice medicine legally. When the GMC withdrew recognition from Indian medical schools, Indian graduates were hardly better situated than Pakistani graduates affected by the retraction of reciprocity in 1972. The government of India preferred that its medical graduates, who were trained at the nation's expense, remain home to deliver health care to its vast underserved population. In raising the opportunity costs associated with migration, the hurdles linked to temporary registration complemented this position, though clearly for different reasons. TRAB imposed an additional hurdle for appointments in the hospital service. The five-year maximum period on the temporary register ensured not only Britain's access to Indian doctors' labor, but also that their stay would be for a limited duration. The choices available to them were accordingly constrained: return to India or migrate elsewhere.

The vulnerability of Indian doctors was an open secret. Officials in the FCO were so comfortable with the overseas committee's recommendation that they went so far as to urge the GMC not to defer acting despite possible protests from its counterpart, the India Council of Medicine, or from affected doctors. Neither were officials in the DHSS worried about any adverse impact. The large numbers of Indian doctors on the waiting list for a clinical attachment ensured that the staffing needs of the NHS would be filled for the foreseeable future. Believing that the Merrison Report would confirm the stereotype of Indian doctors as far less accomplished than domestic graduates, DHSS advised timing the public announcement of the withdrawal of recognition from Indian medical schools to occur after the publication of the final report. In short, the Merrison Report served more as political window dressing for public consumption rather than spurring the GMC decision to revise access to the register without changing the law.

Ending Reciprocity Informally: Withdrawing Recognition from Indian Medical Schools

In a little over a year, the newly established overseas committee of the GMC completed its review of eighty-two qualifications from medical schools in reciprocating countries.[1] Regarded as equivalent to the medical education in the United Kingdom, these qualifications entitled overseas medical graduates to full registration or unrestricted rights to practice medicine. The committee recommended the continuation of recognition for university medical degrees granted in Australia, Canada, Hong Kong, Malaysia, Malta, New Zealand, Singapore, the West Indies and South Africa. Apart from these countries, degrees from two others were still under consideration, namely Burma and Uganda. But the committee's recommendation to withdraw recognition from medical schools in India was by far the most consequential. India stood out from other reciprocating countries with fifty-two medical degrees recognized for full registration, which accounted for 63 percent of the total of 82.

The recommendation to withdraw recognition from Indian medical schools was not a surprise. Even before the review was completed, Draper doubted that the India Medical Council would "be prepared to afford the necessary facilities, and even if visits were permitted the reports hereafter might not be favorable."[2] The Indian Medical Council replied minimally to requests for information about Indian medical colleges. In reference to whether schools were in compliance with its regulations or recommendations concerning the minimal admissions of one hundred students or the education and training level for visiting physician or surgeon appointments, the council responded in general terms that their recommendations were "'by and large' or 'more or less' complied with."[3] Its reports of the periodic inspections were not made available, nor did the GMC's request to inspect elicit even a reply. Withdrawal of recognition was tied to the new testing regime then under development for temporary registration. Rather than assuming that Indian medical graduates were part of a common professional culture of British medicine, their training and experience would now have to be validated for practice in Britain. At most, their qualifications, provided they passed the TRAB test, would entitle them to temporary registration.[4]

Draper consulted relevant government offices. Neither the Minister of Health and of Foreign and Commonwealth Affairs nor their associated departments or offices raised objections to the proposed recommendation. They stressed instead the presentation of the decision to the public in ways that would not unduly provoke India or damage the credibility of Indian doctors employed in the health service. To be sure, government support for the recommendation reflected the degree to which the presence of overseas doctors had become politicized. It no less reflected the structural power of Britain as a recipient nation and India's weakness as a donor nation lacking the ability to effectively control the migration of its medical graduates. A Department of Health study, which formed part of a background briefing to ministers, concluded that the effect of withdrawal would not seriously affect Britain's capacity to fill its manpower needs with overseas doctors. Underlying this confidence was the existence of a large number of Indian-trained doctors on the waiting list for clinical attachment posts.[5] These doctors were a self-selected group of Indian medical graduates who expressed an interest in working in the health service and studying in Britain. Critical to this department was the date that withdrawal was to be enacted: "GMC officials have commented informally that the proposals will not be completely retrospective, but how far back the Council will go is uncertain." Based on a sample of doctors already on the waiting list who qualified before January 1975 and were eligible for full registration, the study estimated that "the potential supply would cover projected requirements to the end of the decade, one or two years 'retrospection' would still leave an adequate reserve." The supply would be augmented by doctors who passed the TRAB examination. The study asserted that "it is too early to predict how many will eventually be processed annually by that system, or what the failure rate will be, but there should be some Indian in-put to swell the reserve of Indians eligible for full registration."[6]

Even though the study was optimistic about the consequences of withdrawal, it emphasized the need to present the decision in ways that did not discourage Indian doctors from pursuing employment in Britain. In the context of the rising demand in the world for trained doctors, Britain was not the only destination. "In the future Arab oil states and Iran, both nearer than Britain, may prove more attractive to Indian doctors. Medical immigration may decline because of economic circumstances."[7] Both to retain the interest of doctors on the waiting list and encourage prospective graduates, the study outlined steps that the GMC along with the DHSS would undertake to minimize the change in the nature of the relationship between the Indian medical profession and Britain. These steps included "careful presentation to Indian medical schools" and "similar presentation for use in any necessary dealings with Indian doctors, e.g. in the attachment scheme or through Foreign and Commonwealth Office channels."[8]

Like the DHSS, the FCO was more concerned with the politics of the recommendation than its merits. Its views were based on the assessment of the British High Commissioner of India (BHCI) and the Southeast Asia Department. Writing on behalf of the BHCI, W. K. K. White anticipated some "cries of anguish and rage in India both from the professional organizations and from the media," but he was not sure about whether the Indian government would take a position. He did not expect the government to come to the defense of the GMC. Still, the uncertainty about what the official response might be was construed to underscore the government's complicity in permitting the proliferation of medical colleges and graduates without sufficient oversight. The lax oversight forced the GMC to take action. "We recognize that embarrassment on the Indian side, deriving from a recognition of the essential rightness of the GMC decision, might lead them to play down publicity which in the last analysis only redound to their own discredit." In the event of a "public row," White did not think any quarrel would adversely affect long-term relations with India and certainly did not justify "arguing that the GMC should not act as proposed."[9]

White sketched out the political management of the decision in ways meant to diminish the scale of protest. Controlling the presentation of information was critical in not putting the government in a defensive position. He stressed that it was better for the government "to be informed by us, rather than be left to find out through their own Medical Council or disgruntled doctors." But timing was no less important in determining when to inform the Ministry of External Affairs for the same reason: "Presumably the GMC does not want the IMC [Indian Medical Council] to start a row before the GMC have arrived at their decision, and it is presumably not for us to betray the GMC's confidences." White therefore proposed formal notification once the decision was made by the GMC but suggested outlining the rationale informally in advance. In providing advance warning, he emphasized "professional and technical grounds" for the decision by the GMC. Any questions about the merits would be directed to the respective national councils. "We would not be prepared to discuss the merits of the case, but would say, in reply to any disposition to do so on the MEA's part, that these were professional questions, which only the Indian Medical Council and the General Medical Council could profitably discuss."[10]

Given the level of ministerial support, the Privy Council for its part raised no objections. Writing on behalf of the council, N. E. Leigh echoed the British High Commission in India when emphasizing the need for consistency. "It is considered desirable that a final decision on this matter should be made at the Council's meeting, and subsequently adhered to. Any suggestions of further delay in which to seek new evidence, or further debate, or a 'period of grace,' could it is felt only lead to embarrassment."[11] The public presentation of the decision was no less important for the council. "Finally, Their Lordships attach great importance to the way in which the change of policy is presented both to the Indian Medical Council and in this country, and I understand that arrangements have been made for this aspect of the matter to be discussed at an early meeting between yourself and officials of the Foreign and Commonwealth Office and the Department of Health and Social Security."[12]

The timing of the scheduled May 22 meeting of the GMC to discuss and adopt the Overseas Committee's recommendation was calculated for maximum effect. It took place a month after the publication of the Merrison Report. This report, which was the culmination of nearly two years of work, devoted an entire chapter to the registration of overseas-trained medical graduates. Even before the report's publication on April 15, it was an open secret that the contents of the chapter would be highly critical of the registration system. Many of the deficiencies were well-known to the GMC and certainly informed the steps undertaken to tighten up the review of medical schools and testing for temporary registration. A submission to ministers anticipated that the report would be critical of the "GMC's previous complaisance about the problem of the standard of overseas doctors," but added that the commission "will commend the line that they are now taking."[13] Although the report did not specifically address the withdrawal of recognition then under consideration, it was hoped that the evidence presented about the competency of overseas-trained doctors would minimize the reaction in India to the announcement on May 22. Nigel Sharp added hopefully, "By this time, however, we hope that the Merrison Report will have been published which may be helpful in dealing with any criticism which arises over India."[14]

The Merrison Committee Report and Recommendations, 1973–75

The principal purpose of the Merrison Committee focused on the regulation of the medical profession. But its membership underscored the mission of regulation: public safety. Its members portrayed British medicine as a public good rather than narrowly defined set of interest groups. This attitude extended from the commission's chair A. W. Merrison, vice chancellor of Bristol University and fellow of the Royal Society, to the other fourteen members. They included representatives from the medical profession, though none from either organized medicine or the London-based elite royal professional colleges. Instead, the Royal Colleges of Nursing, General Practitioners and Psychiatrists, and the British Postgraduate Medical Federation were represented. These bodies formed an important part of the postwar occupational landscape, but they were not formally represented on the GMC even though they were directly or indirectly affected by its decisions. Several senior consultants and general practitioners based in cities outside of London and England, including Hull, Leicestershire, and Aberdeen, augmented the number of members with occupational ties to British medicine. At the same time, representatives from the university and wider community rounded out the committee. They included a vice chancellor and scientist, a barrister and member of the bench for the Isle of Man, a writer, the president of the Council of Industrial Tribunals in Scotland, and the secretary of the General Whitney Council for the Health Services of Great Britain.[15]

Even as the composition of the commission aspired to be broadly representative of the profession and the public alike, one omission was noteworthy: overseas-trained doctors. This omission was not new. Neither the previous commissions on postwar medical manpower (1955) and medical education (1968) nor the joint BMA and GMC working groups (1970–71) included overseas-trained doctors. This omission did not reflect indifference per se, but rather the ways in which national medicine masked the imperial and postimperial nature of British medicine. Rather than being set apart, overseas-trained doctors on the register formed an integral part of the coherent unit that was British medicine. As provided for in the Medical Acts and Amendments, overseas doctors with recognized qualifications from reciprocating countries were entitled to practice medicine without restrictions in the United Kingdom. In theory, at least, their professional integration minimized differences and the need for specific representation. Among the list of names of the 111 professional and medical bodies from which the committee solicited written and in-person evidence, none referred to overseas-trained doctors in general or even to those who were fully registered or temporarily registered. Alone among the 49 individuals who gave evidence, Christopher Terrell, an engineer, discussed the plight of temporarily registered doctors. It is noteworthy that he did so not as a doctor, but as the husband of Victoria Terrell.[16]

Yet the structure and rhetoric of the report reinforced the suspicion about overseas doctors and the need for greater scrutiny. Where six of the seven chapters of the report referred to neutral-sounding processes of regulation, such as registration and education, fitness to practice, and discipline, overseas doctors were set apart in a chapter devoted to them as a particular problem within British medicine. As the introduction made clear, this special attention underscored their inherent liminality within British medicine as an essential source of labor but one that threatened to undermine it: "It is no exaggeration to say that the present level of care provided by the NHS itself would have collapsed along ago without the crucial contribution of overseas doctors."

At the same time, the scale of their contributions posed a threat to the credibility of the NHS. Evidence and testimony that questioned the capacity of overseas doctors to practice medicine in the United Kingdom troubled the committee. The committee framed its work as a type of reclamation project, one that sought to restore confidence in British medicine by clarifying membership within its boundaries chiefly through modifying the system of registration. The global character of British medicine would remain, but the doubts about the professional competency of overseas doctors would be eliminated. The committee stated that "this is obviously a matter of concern to the public who may be treated by overseas doctors, to members of the medical profession whose successful practice will often depend on colleagues' competence, and to overseas practitioners themselves whose effectiveness as doctors may be reduced by doubts about the value of their qualifications."[17]

The report situated overseas doctors in relation to the British nation as the site for the social production of doctors. The category of "overseas" rendered them, at best, a means to supplement the domestic supply of doctors or, at worse, a threat to national norms and public safety. As a result, the globalization of British medicine was framed as a product of recent events and not in its historical context. The committee report said, "The first [question] is the extent to which the GMC should depart from the means which it uses of assuring itself of the quality of doctors in this country—namely, acceptance of the assessment of the candidate's medical school—and operate [*sic*] assessment of individuals' knowledge." Decolonization diluted the special bonds of British medicine, the report suggested, while the successor states of the empire pursued medical education that related to their national needs and interests. "Clearly, the GMC has not, and can never have, the same intimate knowledge of overseas medical schools as it has of the medical schools of the country."[18] The report's concern with the competency of the GMC to assess fitness to practice masked how the structure of imperial rule—not the medical training in the United Kingdom per se—had been the basis of the territorial jurisdiction of British medicine and the privileges enjoyed by domestic white male medical graduates in the world. The decolonization of medicine produced heterogeneity while reshaping an imperial profession into a national one. In the postwar era, a medical degree from India ceased to be a recognized sign of membership in the fraternity of British medicine and thereby necessitated greater policing of the boundaries of national medicine.

The evidence for the unsuitability of overseas doctors practicing medicine in the United Kingdom was not based on their medical training per se, but rather on the comparative performance of fully registered overseas-trained doctors on the fellowship examination for the Royal Colleges of General Medicine and Psychiatry.[19] In general, possessing a fellowship diploma represented an important career milestone. It conferred membership among senior practitioners whose experience and expertise exceeded the minimum needed to practice medicine. Long regarded as a mark of distinction, the diploma became expected as one moved up the pyramid-shaped career structure of the NHS. But eligibility to sit for the examination, much less passing it, was challenging given the informal nature of hospital-based training. As elite members of the profession, hospital consultants sat atop the pyramid of the medical staff. They regulated the social production of specialists. Consultants selected incumbents for junior and more senior appointments that functioned as the training ground for future fellows and consultants. In addition, obtaining relevant course work presented its own challenge. Greater London offered an extensive range of specialty schools, which the British Postgraduate Medical Federation had coordinated since 1935. This was not the case for doctors who were situated in remote (rural or urban) areas or who staffed hospitals that were not affiliated with medical schools.[20] While these challenges affected UK-trained doctors, overseas-trained doctors faced additional hurdles. They lacked access to informal networks, which were crucial to secure hospital appointments in prestigious medical and surgical specialties. Constrained financial means were an additional factor in channeling overseas doctors into appointments in nonteaching hospitals and less prestigious specialties. In psychiatry, for example, South Asian doctors in 1972 accounted for 60 percent of registrars, 34 percent of senior registrars, and 16 percent of consultants.

The report scarcely acknowledged these structural hurdles in discussing the performance of overseas doctors on higher qualifications in psychiatry or general medicine. Whether presented in tabular or narrative format, the data drew an unfavorable distinction between domestic and overseas medical graduates. To underscore the point, the report disaggregated overseas doctors, separating those from former white settler colonies (or the old Commonwealth) and the subcontinent (India, Pakistan and Bangladesh) and the United Arab Republic. The first group and the latter two yielded pass rates of 81 percent and 47 percent respectively. As if the low pass rate was not enough, the report also emphasized the overrepresentation of overseas doctors in hospital psychiatry units. The implication was clear enough in terms of patient safety: the most vulnerable received care at the hands of the least qualified. The narrative of failure was the same for general medicine. The committee regarded the pass rate of just three out of forty-nine on the Royal College of General Practitioners fellowship examination for overseas doctors as "disturbing," echoing the view of the college itself. Although the report provided the same level of detail about the representation of overseas doctors in general medicine within the hospital service, the comparison to the performance of United Kingdom graduates made the conclusion inescapable. British doctors were better, and patients were in safer hands.[21]

The committee complemented its quantitative analysis of comparative pass rates with qualitative evidence. Rather than seeking out such evidence, the report noted, "we could not fail to be aware of a widespread conviction that the standard of overseas educated doctors allowed to practice in this country is lower than that of home-educated doctors." This conviction was not only reflected in the letters to the editor in the *British Medical Journal* but also surfaced in oral evidence. The report of the testimony from the Royal College of Nursing painted a portrait of overseas practitioners whose cultural differences were so total that they damaged the integrity of British medicine. Their limited command of English minimized the value of the telephone or the utility of hospital technology while raising the risk of inaccurate "medical instructions." In psychiatric hospitals, the misunderstanding of colloquial expressions used by patients jeopardized the accuracy of clinical diagnosis and treatment. "An example was given," said the report, "of the doctor from abroad who interpreted the use of colloquialism by the patient as a sign of confusion and disorientation." In short, overseas doctors were cultural aliens who attempted to practice medicine in an alien culture. "The ethical principles and cultural background peculiar to the United Kingdom give rise to a great deal of difficulty for doctors from certain countries where values and principles are different."[22]

It is noteworthy that the report used neither the term Indian nor overseas, nor did it even specify their registration status (full or temporary). In light of the discussion of comparative pass rates, it was still a relatively easy inference for the reader to apply the general comments to overseas-trained doctors from India. Crucial to the credibility of the critique was the assumption that the nurses that staffed the hospital service were overwhelmingly British, even though the health service relied on overseas-born or -trained nurses.[23] To the extent that nurses were compelled to second-guess not just the meaning of the language used by overseas doctors but also the appropriateness of medical directions, the report implied, the hierarchy of roles and authority within the hospital was weakened to the detriment of patient health.

The committee drew the conclusion that the educational standards of overseas doctors were not equivalent to UK standards: "We believe there are substantial numbers of overseas doctors whose skill and the care they offer to patients fall below that generally acceptable in this country, and it is at least possible that there are some who should not have been registered at all." Nor did it entertain much confidence in those who were professionally competent to meet the "bedside test," that is to say, the capacity to communicate with patients and engage in appropriate professional behavior. "Even where an overseas doctor is fully knowledgeable and articulate in the professional field," the reported declared, "his difficulty in communicating with patients in nonmedical terms may constitute a major barrier to his integration into medical practice in this country." In short, overseas doctors lacked the cultural competency necessary to be effective practitioners in Britain. "It would be surprising if doctors from overseas did not lack knowledge of the operation of the NHS, did not find difficulty in understanding the significance of the euphemisms and colloquialisms which for many patients are their most accurate means of expression, and even more surprising if they could easily come to grips with the variety of dialects they may encounter. This will particularly be the case where the graduate comes from a country where English is not spoken or where the use of English as a teaching language is being discontinued."[24]

This state of affairs amounted to a dereliction of the GMC's duty. In a stinging rebuke, the committee declared "we believe that this unsatisfactory situation is principally to be attributed to a willingness on the part of the GMC to allow its duty as the protector of medical standards to be compromised by the manpower requirements of the NHS."[25] The burden of responsibility did not rest wholly with the GMC. The imperative to meet the staffing needs of the DHSS subverted the function of registration as a safeguard for medical standards. Even the department's expectation that overseas doctors "whose medical education and ability are of an appropriate standard and character for work in the NHS" not be deterred or impeded due to excessive conditions was regarded as admission of the toleration of a double standard.[26] "It allows for the possibility that in the United Kingdom the educational standards are and should be, as high as, or higher than anywhere in the world, but that, provided an overseas doctor is competent at a reasonable and appropriate standard for a junior hospital post, he should be allowed in by the GMC, even though it may be uncertain whether his country's educational standards are as high as ours." Having created a straw argument, the committee rejected it. "We do not accept that doctors in the

British Isles are trained to an unnecessarily high standard—and we doubt whether the assertion of the contrary by the Health Department would be accepted to be a disinterested comment. It is not for us to judge the ethics of a service which relies on a substantial supply of doctors from countries which are themselves seriously short of medical services."[27]

In exposing the effects of the globalization of British medicine, the committee certainly assigned responsibility. It also commended the responsiveness of the GMC. Here the report endorsed the council's recommendations to tighten up procedures for the registration of overseas-trained doctors, relying on a mix of its existing authority and suggestions for amending legislation at a future time. The latter would include replacing temporary registration with limited registration and providing for the full registration of distinguished doctors at the discretion of the council. Under the former, overseas doctors seeking admission to the temporary registrar would be required to pass the TRAB examination for clinical and English-language competency.[28] In principle the committee welcomed the elimination of full registration for medical graduates with recognized qualifications from reciprocating countries. Rather than being an instrument to promote a uniform standard of British medicine, the committee argued, reciprocity subverted it. The committee concurred with the purpose of registration as articulated by the GMC: "The system of registration should be directed to the maintenance of standards in this country, and the presence or absence of privileges of practice in the country of provenance is irrelevant to this purpose."[29]

Furthermore, the mechanism for scrutinizing overseas senior medical professionals or specialists provided for differential treatment of doctors from nonreciprocating countries. Under proposed amending legislation, the committee supported granting discretionary authority to the GMC to grant full registration to "distinguished" doctors. The safeguards associated with the GMC's exercise of discretionary authority created hurdles for overseas doctors, especially those who were educated, trained, and practiced in new Commonwealth countries. The committee urged that British medical institutions—royal colleges, medical faculties, and professional associations, among others—vet and recommend overseas doctors as part of an alternative path to full registration. While this step supplemented the evaluation of the GMC, its very nature advantaged overseas doctors who were integrated within professional or specialist networks, including doctors from Europe and the United States.[30]

While doctors from Europe and the United States would be granted registration on the strength of their reputation in the United Kingdom under proposed amending legislation, all overseas doctors seeking specialist registration would be required to obtain general registration as a precondition. Fully registered doctors would thereafter satisfy the conditions of experience and pass the relevant accrediting examination to be a registered specialist in the United Kingdom.[31] At first sight, the committee's suggestion appeared to clarify the respective roles and responsibilities of the GMC and specialist bodies. Under the existing Medical Act, in theory overseas doctors entitled to full registration would not be directly affected. But they would be affected in the event that the GMC withdrew recognition from their qualifications. Withdrawal of recognition would mean that affected overseas doctors who sought specialist registration could only satisfy the condition of primary qualification if they requalified in Britain. This placed them in the identical position of "distinguished" doctors. But as noted above, the provision that the committee proposed for accommodating doctors who lacked recognized primary qualifications advantaged those who were known or familiar to British practitioners and specialists.

The discussion of overseas doctors was only part of a much larger report that related to the regulation of the profession. Medical education and registration, fitness to practice and discipline, and composition, financing, and structure of the council were the key themes of the report. Animating the themes and associated recommendations were a set of principles that emphasized the continued role of an independent body regulating the medical profession; the expansion of interest groups, that is, the professional colleges and universities, the profession, and members of the lay community; and the clarification of roles and responsibilities between the GMC, the wider medical profession, and the public. For the most part, the recommendations called for consolidating the role of the GMC through greater coordination of all stages of education and the creation and dedicated oversight of a new register for specialists; refining the machinery for discipline and fitness to practice that balanced the right of registered doctors to practice medicine and the interests of the public through the establishment of a health committee for sick doctors and the adoption and dissemination of best practices; and expanding the membership of the council to ninety-eight, including forty-four nominated representatives (thirty-four from educational institutions and ten lay members by the Crown), and fifty-four elected at large from within the profession. The committee was acutely conscious of the scale of the task that it set before the government, the profession, and the public alike. Aware of the momentum created by the inquiry and the risk of delay in implementing the recommendations in their entirety, the committee called for prompt action. "Our report will take many years to implement and we think further delay on this account would be unacceptable. We hope we have suggested a system of regulation which would be appropriate at least for the rest of the century; that ought not to be the excuse for not getting on with the job."[32]

Published in April, the Merrison Report was well received. "A Good Report" was the title of a leading article in the *British Medical Journal*.[33] *The Lancet* noted optimistically that the report "has the makings of a landmark as massive as the first Medical Act of 1858."[34] At the same time, the retrospective criticism for the past and prospective praise for future arrangements for the registration of overseas doctors introduced a discordant strain in the reception. For the *BMJ*, the labors of the Merrison Committee vindicated its long criticism of the inadequacy, if not failure, of the GMC and the Department of Health and Social Security to protect the public. "For the first time an authoritative body has had the courage to state that the N.H.S. has been kept going by employing overseas doctors whose skill and the care they offer to patients fall below that generally acceptable in this country," a leader defiantly declared.[35] While the GMC accepted the negative judgment of medical education overseas, it objected to the criticism that it was responsible for them or that patient safety was at risk. Conversely, the endorsement of its proposals was presented as vindication of its role in regulating access to the medical market.[36]

Underlying the reception was the unquestioned assumption that the English-language and clinical competence of overseas doctors was suspect and would continue to be so unless corrective action was taken. *The Lancet* anticipated that "the new examinations to be introduced later this year by the G.M.C. will reduce the number of overseas doctors entering the N.H.S.—for if they are to be of any value the tests must exclude those whose English comprehension or medical competence is below the minimum required of a British medical graduate." Obliquely acknowledging the racism that inflected the blanket characterization of overseas doctors as substandard, the leader was hopeful that TRAB would render the racial characteristics of overseas doctors irrelevant in the judgment of the profession and the public. "In time they should free the many excellent overseas doctors practicing here of the blanket criticism that the minority of incompetent have provoked."[37] The leader did not specify the length of time when a formal assessment would render all other considerations inconsequential. In the meantime, the competency of overseas doctors would remain subject to racial stereotypes of fitness to practice medicine in the United Kingdom.

The consensus of British medicine that formed behind the Merrison Report added momentum to the decision of the GMC to withdraw recognition from medical schools in India. Indeed, within a month of the release of the report, the council considered and accepted the recommendation of the Overseas Committee. In light of the consultations with relevant government departments—not to mention the Privy Council, this decision was hardly a surprise. The timing of the decision afforded the GMC the collective endorsement of British medicine. The decision to withdraw recognition did not deny entry to all doctors from India. Rather it redefined the conditions under which they could participate in British medicine. Indian doctors who possessed recognized qualifications before the May 22 date would be eligible for full registration. All others unless exempted would be eligible for temporary registration after passing the TRAB examination and completing a period of attachment.

Neither the Merrison Report nor the withdrawal of recognition escaped criticism. After the report's publication, letters in the medical press shortly began appearing that were critical and at least complicated the committee's analysis and conclusion about overseas doctors. Troubled by the rhetoric, S. K. Roy characterized the report as being more a political document than one designed to improve standards. Far from being disinterested, Roy characterized the committee as acting as little more than "prosecutor, jury, and judge of the overseas doctors, who now constitute 16% of general practitioners and 40% of junior doctors in Britain." In a not so veiled reference to the anti-immigration rhetoric within and outside of organized medicine, Roy denounced the committee for giving "into the pressure groups who wish to restrict the immigration of doctors. It is well known that there has always been a vocal group who felt that their bargaining position was weakened by the presence of overseas doctors here."[38]

The medical press commentary continued when the GMC withdrew recognition from Indian medical schools. Much of it historicized the contingent place of Indian doctors in postwar British medicine. "When the N.H.S. was in danger of collapse, Asian doctors were not only welcomed and were encouraged to come and work here. Now they are being humiliated in a general attack, though a big majority has faithfully and efficiently served the N.H.S.," wrote D. R. Prem, president of the Standing Conference of Asian Organizations in the United Kingdom.[39] For S. K. Roy, the "resentment and bitterness" in the general profession was less about standards than the politics of the NHS. Indian doctors served as convenient scapegoats for the profession, just as they were a convenient source of labor for the Department of Health. "In the view of British doctors and their organization this has frustrated their hopes of achieving better remuneration and conditions of service." Roy added. "No country should have to rely on foreign doctors, but let us not make the mistake of inferring that the words of 'overseas' and 'inferior' are synonymous."[40] Dr. R. K. Gulati, a general practitioner in Watford, Hertfordshire, deplored the negative publicity about overseas doctors. Gulati regarded the "decline in patient faith and confidence in general practitioners and junior hospital doctors" as little more than an excuse for the limited opportunities for advanced training. "Most overseas doctors in the U.K. try to further their knowledge and experience. There are no adequate postgraduate training programs. Overseas doctors hardly get a chance to work in teaching hospitals."[41] Conversely, Vinay Bhushan captured the burden that confronted overseas doctors as competency became racialized. "I have quite an experience in satisfying examiners in this country—not only examiners but consultants with whom I have worked and, more importantly, my patients. But thanks to the media of television and press suddenly I am a doctor who does not know English and has no basic medical knowledge and technical ability. Would somebody tell me how to tell people at large that I am an exception? Should I carry my testimonials, diplomas, etc. with me all the time?"[42] Bhushan's rhetorical question captured the double standard for overseas doctors in the United Kingdom. The effect of the discourse and institutional structures, which defined British medicine as homogenous, cast suspicion upon overseas doctors because of their manifest heterogeneity. Neither testimonial nor diploma could change the racial difference of overseas doctors practicing medicine in Britain.

Conclusion

The final report of the Merrison committee did not mark change but continuity in the redefinition of overseas doctors within British medicine. Its recommendations endorsed the strategy that the GMC had pursued since the late 1960s to narrow the portal of entry into the domestic medical profession. Under growing pressure from the medical profession and the government, the council launched both an unprecedented review of medical schools whose medical qualifications were recognized for full registration and the development of a new assessment instrument for temporary registration. The focus of these activities was India. It was the largest source of overseas doctors in the NHS out of thirteen reciprocating countries in the Commonwealth. Given their presence, India doctors became a convenient target for a racialized discourse about professional and cultural competency to practice medicine in the United Kingdom. Withdrawing recognition from India was a foregone conclusion in the GMC even before the review was complete. Access to the domestic medical market was limited to the temporary register only after passing the newly mandated TRAB examination.

Withdrawing recognition from Indian medical training institutions addressed the political problem of Indian doctors in the United Kingdom without closing off a critical source of labor for the NHS. It is for these reasons that the Privy Council approved the recommendation. Neither the DHSS nor the Foreign and Commonwealth Office raised objections. The unflagging desire of Indian doctors to practice medicine in Britain was sufficiently robust to withstand any disruption. Those who did travel to Britain were vulnerable precisely because they were a globalized labor force. They could neither look to their government for assistance nor challenge the conditions for admissions to the register. They ceased being an integral part of the fraternity of British medicine. Instead, they were adequately trained doctors who supplemented the staffing in the hospital service and practiced medicine under the direct supervision of senior, largely white and male British medical professionals and authorities. To be sure, the Merrison Committee was highly critical of the GMC's oversight of the register as it related to the registration of overseas doctors. The report at the same time welcomed and endorsed the council's steps to narrow access to the register. Ultimately, the structural subordination of overseas doctors to British medical graduates helped to restore the credibility of the GMC to regulate the profession.

Conclusion

Overseas Doctors Needed, but Not Wanted

Three years after the Merrison Committee submitted its final report, Parliament passed the 1978 Medical Act. In reference to the registration of overseas doctors, the provisions of the act reflected more continuity than change. The GMC's oversight of the register remained intact. The Medical Act's scheduled termination of reciprocity on December 1, 1980, came as no real surprise. The retraction of reciprocity from Pakistan in 1972 and the subsequent withdrawal of recognition of Indian medical qualifications a year later anticipated this provision of the legislation while underscoring the politically conditional relationship of overseas doctors to British medicine.[1] The terms of access to the medical market were no more surprising. Overseas doctors were now required to pass the Professional and Linguistic Assessment Board (PLAB) examination, which replaced the TRAB examination. For those who passed the PLAB, the right to practice medicine was still subject to restrictions regarding length and place even after the category of temporary registration was replaced by the category of limited registration.

The act enhanced the authority of the GMC over registration even as the relationship of overseas doctors to British medicine became more contingent. After years of lobbying, the council now enjoyed discretionary power to specify the duration and clinical assignment for doctors who were admitted under limited registration. It was also empowered to grant full registration to those overseas doctors who satisfied the necessary medical qualifications and clinical experience. In sum, the act formalized what postwar British medicine had become: a globalized medical profession that was stratified between domestic and overseas graduates, one largely white and permanent and the other largely nonwhite and transient.

As I have argued in this book, the inequitable treatment of overseas doctors of color was not so much a historical accident of the postwar period but rather a result of the careful political management of the national and imperial boundaries that historically circumscribed British medicine. Since

1858, the medical register had fortified these boundaries, creating a space for the growth and consolidation of British medicine as a social institution. Admission to the register—a crucial step toward success in the British medical occupation—was tied to the possession of a medical qualification from designated university and nonuniversity licensing bodies in the United Kingdom. This relationship shaped the contours of British medicine in several ways. It constrained the growth of a domestic profession long regarded to be overcrowded and opened the empire as a destination for the surplus supply of doctors for private practice and government service. At the same time, the largely tacit obstacles that nonwhite colonial subjects and British white women faced in obtaining a medical qualification were no less consequential. The medical profession collectively privileged domestic graduates over colonial graduates and masked the perpetuation of gender and racial hierarchies that defined the British profession. Indeed, by the turn of the twentieth century, the modern identity of British medicine as an imperial profession was complete. It was a normatively white and male profession and enjoyed a relatively stable size in relation to the general population.

This identity shaped the relationship of overseas-trained doctors to British medicine. In opening and closing the register in the twentieth century, the GMC regulated access to the medical market in response to the labor requirements of Britain. Britain supplemented its supply of domestically produced doctors by recruiting doctors from reciprocating white settler Dominions during World War I. It augmented this supply during World War II by providing for the temporary registration of doctors trained in allied, belligerent, and neutral countries. These efforts, which mitigated pressure on the domestic profession, did not fundamentally jeopardize the identity of British medicine. The very temporary nature of the wartime exigency limited their use. Whether responding to the needs of the mother country or the Allied cause, these doctors reflected the social image of British medicine. They were predominately white and male. Both the nature and terms of their registration assumed that they would return to their countries of origins at the end of the war rather than settle and practice medicine in the United Kingdom.

Yet, the very vehicle—the register—that limited access to British medicine during the world wars operated as an existential threat to its social identity in the postwar period. The domestic production of doctors remained unchanged from interwar levels. Expanding Britain's supply of doctors was not a particularly high priority of postwar planning until the mid-1960s. In the meantime, Britain and the GMC, among other entities, encouraged overseas-trained doctors, particularly from the Commonwealth, to pursue postgraduate training in the United Kingdom. This encouragement served multiple purposes, ranging from projecting Britain's influence into the world as a postimperial power and strengthening ties among newly independent Commonwealth countries to meeting the labor needs of the hospital service of the National Health Service (NHS). The presence of overseas doctors in the hospital service was tolerated in large part because of restrictions on the duration and place of practice for those who were admitted to the temporary register. This was not the case for overseas doctors from reciprocating nonwhite new Commonwealth countries such as India and Pakistan. Together these countries not only became the leading exporters of overseas doctors on the temporary register, they also accounted for a disproportionate number of overseas doctors that were granted unrestricted rights to practice medicine or full registration. They became the focal point of racial anxieties about the nature of postwar British medicine.

In response to the globalization of British medicine, critics of registration decried the fact that doctors from nonreciprocating European countries were restricted to the temporary register whereas those from reciprocating countries were granted full registration only because of the historical accident of imperialism. This comparison drew an unfavorable distinction between doctors from Europe and those who were overwhelmingly from the nonwhite countries in the Commonwealth. This implicit racial binary quickly became an explicit staple of the discourse within and outside of the profession. Crucial to this transition was the meaning assigned to the migration of domestic medical graduates. Several hundred graduates annually left Britain in search of more lucrative career opportunities in the United States or in countries of the "old" Commonwealth. Critics of the NHS viewed these graduates' mobility not as part of a fundamental feature of the modern profession, but rather as an indictment of the inadequate opportunities within the service. Conversely, overseas doctors, who supplemented the flat domestic production of medical graduates, were portrayed in the medical press as suspect. Rather than representing British medicine's imperial legacy, their training outside of the United Kingdom raised doubts about their competency to practice medicine. This racialized view of competence was epitomized by the concern over overseas doctors' ability to speak English in clinical settings, which reinforced fears about patient safety and doubts about their capacity to fully assimilate into British medicine. In perpetuating the fictive homogeneity of British medicine, the GMC adopted or approved measures that rendered overseas doctors little more than adjuncts to the domestic profession.

As the twentieth century came to a close, the position of overseas doctors—both those who were on the limited register and those on the full register—became more insecure rather than less. The portals to the register progressively narrowed as an effect of a national self-sufficiency policy that increased the number of domestic medical graduates while limiting the admission of overseas doctors to those who had at least completed the equivalent of a preregistration or internship year. From 1978 onward, the GMC exempted on average 35 percent of applicants from the mandatory PLAB test based on their prearranged selection for approved training programs in the United Kingdom.[2] But in 1983 the exemption policy was revised. The threshold now included the completion of a minimum of two years of postgraduate training (one in a specialty) or appointment at the registrar level. By 1995 the GMC ended the exemption policy altogether. In the meantime, the employment status of overseas doctors became even more problematic.[3] The 1978 Act did not mandate that overseas doctors possess a work permit while employed in a NHS approved training post. In practice, any extension of permit-free status or extension of a work permit was subject to the discretion of the Home Office.[4] As many overseas doctors later discovered, a denial of an extension request was often accompanied by an order to leave the country. Although a fifth permit-free year was added and increased to six in 1997 with the approval of the student's postgraduate dean, this accommodation only reinforced the contingent nature of their presence.[5] By the end of the century, these changes would culminate in a government directive in 2006 that allowed the appointment of an overseas doctor only when a suitable medical graduate from the United Kingdom or a European Union (EU) member country was not available.[6]

The preferential treatment of doctors from EU member states underscored the marginality of overseas doctors, particularly those who obtained full registration. After two previous attempts, Britain's member state application to join the six-country predecessor to the EU, the European Economic Community (EEC), was approved in 1973. In agreeing to the free movement of citizens—including doctors—within the community, Britain accepted the curtailment of the rights of doctors on the register who were trained overseas. This policy negatively impacted fully registered Commonwealth citizens, who were overwhelming South Asian with British nationality. Their only alternative was to requalify in the United Kingdom. This policy and its uneven impact continued as the European Union—the successor to the EEC—expanded to twenty-seven member countries after 1993. Even though fully registered overseas doctors of color are more secure that those on the limited register, their differential treatment highlights a persistent reality: they will never be full members of British medicine. It is unlikely that Britain's decision in June 2016 to leave the European Union will change the perception and experience of overseas doctors. In the twenty-first century as in the twentieth century, they will be needed, but not wanted.

Notes

Introduction

1. Laurence Brockliss, "The Professions and National Identity," in *A Union of Multiple Identities: The British Isles, 1750–1850,* ed. Laurence Brockliss and David Eastwood (Manchester, UK: Manchester University Press, 1997), 18–21.

2. Peter Bartrip, *Themselves Writ Large: The British Medical Association, 1832–1966* (London: BMJ Publishing Group, 1996), 1, 20, 29–34, 41, 50–55.

3. The scholarly literature on the relationship of imperialism and national identity continues to grow. For representative discussions, see Catherine Hall and Sonya Rose, eds., *At Home with Empire: Metropolitan Culture and the Imperial World* (Cambridge: Cambridge University Press, 2006); Philippa Levine, *Prostitution, Race & Politics: Policing Venereal Disease in the British Empire* (London: Routledge, 2003); Rieko Karatani, *Defining British Citizenship: Empire, Commonwealth and Modern Britain* (London: Frank Cass, 2003); Catherine Hall, *Civilising Subjects: Metropole and Colony in the English Imagination, 1830–1867* (Chicago: University of Chicago Press, 2002); Douglas M. Haynes, *Imperial Medicine: Patrick Manson and the Conquest of Tropical Disease* (Philadelphia: University of Pennsylvania Press, 2001); Mrinalini Sinha, *Colonial Masculinity: "The Manly Englishmen" and the "Effeminate Bengali" in the Late Nineteenth Century* (Manchester, UK: Manchester University Press, 1995); and Antoinette Burton, *Burdens of History: British Feminists, Indian Women, and Imperial Culture* (Chapel Hill: University of North Carolina Press, 1994).

4. Douglas M. Haynes, "Victorian Imperialism in the Making of the British Medical Profession: An Argument," in *Decentering Empire: Britain, India and the Transcolonial World,* ed. Durba Ghosh and Dane Kennedy (Hyderabad, India: Orient Longman, 2006), 130–56.

5. On women in modern British medicine, see Ann Digby, *The Evolution of British General Practice* (Oxford: Oxford University Press, 1999); Shirley Roberts, *Sophia Jex-Blake: A Woman Pioneer in Nineteenth Century Medical Reform* (London: Routledge, 1993); and Thomas Bonner, *To the Ends of the Earth: Women's Search for Education in Medicine* (Cambridge, MA: Harvard University Press, 1992). For the relationship of the GMC and the colonial Indian medical profession, see Roger Jeffery, "Recognizing India's Doctors: The Institutionalization of Medical Dependency, 1918–1939," *Modern Asian Studies* 13, no. 2 (April 1979): 301–26. On Jewish medical refugees, see Karola Decker, "Divisions and Diversity: The Complexities of Medical Refuge in Britain, 1933–1948," *Bulletin of the History of Medicine* 77 (2003):

850–73. For a divergent interpretation, see Paul Weindling, "Medical Refugees and the Modernization of British Medicine, 1930–1960," *Social History of Medicine* 22, no. 3 (2009): 489–511.

6. In the twentieth century as in the nineteenth, racial, ethnic, and gender discourses of nation and national belonging articulated a fictive unity through difference. They naturalized racial and gender hierarchies of privilege in a society which in turn required constant policing to mask or reconcile the contradictions between human capacity and individual rights and the structures of inequality within the imperial nation-state.

7. Apart from Karola's study, there has been no sustained study of the use of overseas-trained doctors in World Wars I and II. For an otherwise valuable contribution, see Mark Harrison, *Medicine and Victory: British Military Medicine in the Second World War* (Oxford: Oxford University Press, 2004) and *The Medical War: British Military Medicine and the First World War* (Oxford: Oxford University Press, 2010).

8. See Emma L. Jones and Stephanie J. Snow, *Against the Odds: Black and Minority Ethnic Clinicians and Manchester, 1948 to 2009* (Manchester, UK: Manchester NHS Primary Care Trust, 2010); Andrew Hull and Sanjoy Bhattacharya, "Health Service Sepoys? A Review of the Role of South Asians in the United Kingdom, c. 1947–1980"; and Christopher Kyriakides and Satnam Virdee, "Migrant Labour, Racism and the British National Service," *Ethnicity & Health* 8, no. 4 (November 2003): 283–305; and Karola Decker, "Overseas Doctors: Past and Present," in *Racism in Medicine*, ed. Naaz Coker (London: King's Fund Publishing, 2001), 23–53.

Chapter One

1. On the nexus between medicine, trade, and the empire up to the early nineteenth century, see Richard B. Sheridan, *Doctors and Slaves: A Medical and Demographic History of Slavery in the British West Indies, 1680–1834* (Cambridge: Cambridge University Press, 1985), 42–71; William N. Boog, "Four Monopolies and the Surgeons on London and Edinburgh," *Journal of the History of Medicine* 25, no. 3 (July 1970): 311–22; and James LoGerfo, "Sir William Dolben and 'The Cause of Humanity': The Passage of the Save Trade Regulation Act of 1788," *Eighteenth Century Studies* 6, no. 4 (Summer 1973): 431–52.

2. In the meantime, the expansion of the medical authority, particularly over the working class body, was closely linked to state intervention. See Nadja Durbach, *Bodily Matters: The Anti-vaccination Movement in England, 1853–1907* (Durham, NC: Duke University Press, 2005) and Ruth Richardson, *Death, Dissection and the Destitute* (London: Routledge, 1987).

3. For representative accounts, see Ivan Waddington, *The Medical Profession in the Industrial Revolution* (Dublin: Gill and Macmillan, 1986); Margaret Stacey, *Regulating British Medicine: The General Medical Council* (Chichester, UK: Wiley, 1992), 15–20, and M. Jeanne Peterson, *The Medical Profession in Mid-Victorian London* (Berkeley: University of California Press, 1978), 34–39. More recently, M. J. D. Roberts has examined the process that culminated in the act as a political mediation of lay and professional conceptions of the place of the practitioner in society. See "The Politics

of Professionalization: MPs, Medical Men, and the 1858 Medical Act," *Medical History* 53 (2009): 37–56.

4. Sections 4, 27, 21–35; 46 & 47 Medical Act c. 90. On the relationship of the register to the expansion of the imperial state, see Haynes, "Victorian Imperialism in the Making of the British Medical Profession, 136–38.

5. Sections 3, 4, 6, 10–11, 24; 46 & 47 Medical Act c. 90.

6. Section 19.

7. Sections 13 and 18–24; 46 & 47 Medical Act c. 90.

8. Ibid.

9. Peterson, *The Medical Profession in Mid-Victorian London*, 23–30.

10. Dorothy Porter, *Health, Civilization and the State: A History of Public Health from Ancient to Modern Times* (London: Routledge, 1999), and Dorothy Porter, "Stratification and Its Discontents: Professionalisation and Conflict in British Public Health Services, 1848–1914," in *A History of Education in Public Health*, ed. Elizabeth Fee and Roy Acheson (Oxford: Oxford University Press, 1991), 83–113; M. W. Flinn, "Medical Services under the New Poor Law," in *The New Poor Law in the Nineteenth Century*, ed. Derek Fraser (London: Macmillan, 1976); Jeanne Brand, *Doctors and the State: The British Medical Profession and Government Growth, 1870–1912* (Baltimore: Johns Hopkins University Press, 1965).

11. This estimate is based on the following: 900 in the Army Medical Department, 320 in the Colonial Medical Services, 800 in the Indian Medical Service, and 400 in the Naval Medical Department. Mark Harrison, *Public Heath in British India: Anglo-Indian Preventive Medicine, 1859–1914* (Cambridge: Cambridge University Press, 1994), 6–35; Neil Cantlie, *A History of the Army Medical Department*, vol. 2 (Edinburgh: Churchill Livingstone, 1974), 269–70, 279, 284; "Medical Appointments in the Colonies," *British Medical Journal* 2 (August 28, 1897): 558–59; and Christopher Lloyd and Jack Coulter, *Medicine and the Navy, 1815–1900*, vol. 4 (London: E & S Livingstone, 1963), 10.

12. Although Britain remained a Protestant identified state, Irish Catholic surgeons were able to mediate their imperial and national identities while serving in the Royal Navy in the second half of the nineteenth century. See S. Karly Kehoe, "Accessing Empire: Irish Surgeons and the Royal Navy, 1840–1880," *Social History of Medicine* 26, no. 2 (September 2013): 202–24.

13. Western medical education leading to a registrable qualification—as distinct from training as an auxiliary—was nonexistent in the British West Indies or west Africa until the mid-twentieth century. See Douglas M. Haynes "The Persistence of Privilege: British Medical Qualifications and the Practice of Medicine in the Empire" in *Beyond Sovereignty: Britain, Empire and Transnationalism, c. 1880–1950*, ed. K. Grant, P. Levine, and F. Trentmann (Houndsmills, UK: Palgrave, 2007), 221–27.

14. P. C. Sen Gupta, "Soorjo Coomar Goodeve Chuckerbutty: The First Indian Contributors to Modern Medical Science," *Medical History* 14 (1970): 183–90, and David Arnold, *The New Cambridge History of India*, vol. 3, *Science, Technology and Medicine in Colonial India* (Cambridge: Cambridge University Press, 2000), 61–65.

15. By 1920, one thousand were employed as assistant surgeons in the provincial medical departments and another four thousand as subassistants. Arnold, *India: Science, Technology and Medicine in Colonial India*, 64.

16. Anil Kumar, *Medicine and the Raj: British Medical Policy in India, 1835–1911* (New Delhi: Sage, 1998), 126–31.

17. This division of labor between registered British doctors and nonwhite colonial medical personnel was not confined to India. For others cases see, See Hibba Abugideri, *Gender and the Making of Modern Medicine in Colonial Egypt* (Farnham, UK: Ashgate, 2010), and Heather Bell, *Frontiers of Medicine in the Anglo-Egyptian Sudan, 1899–1940* (Oxford: Clarendon Press, 1999).

18. Adell Patton Jr., *Physicians, Colonial Racism, and Diaspora in West Africa* (Gainesville: University of Florida Press, 1997), 64–73. On the Scottish–West Indian connection, see Sheridan, *Doctors and Slaves,* 55–64.

19. Patton, *Physicians, Colonial Racism, and Diaspora in West Africa,* 74, 78.

20. "The Climate of the West Coast of Africa," *The Lancet* 2 (November 28, 1863): 626.

21. Patton, *Physicians, Colonial Racism, and Diaspora in West Africa,* 93–154. See also T. S. Gale, Official Medical Policy in British West Africa, 1870–1930" (PhD diss., University of London, 1973), 154–206.

22. British Guiana engaged in a similar policy. See Juanita De Barros, "'Spreading Sanitary Enlightenment': Race, Identity, and the Emergence of a Creole Medical Profession in British Guiana," *Journal of British Studies,* 42, no. 2, 2003: 488–96.

23. Patton, *Physicians, Colonial Racism, and Diaspora in West Africa,* 128–31. Other colonial services either explicitly or implicitly adopted this policy. See Anna Crozier, *Practicing Colonial Medicine: The Colonial Medical Service in East Africa* (London: I. B. Tauris, 2007), and Lenore Manderson, *Sickness and the State: Health and Illness in Colonial Malaya, 1870–1940* (Cambridge: Cambridge University Press, 1996).

24. Ann Digby, "'A Medical El Dorado'? Colonial Medical Incomes and Practice at the Cape," *Social History of Medicine* 8, no. 3 (1995): 453–79; James Bradley, Ann Crowther, and Marguerite Dupree, "Mobility and Selection in Scottish University Medical Education, 1858–1886," *Medical History* 40 (1996); Greta Jones, "'Strike out Boldly for the Prizes that are Available to You': Medical Emigration from Ireland, 1870–1905," *Medical History* 54, no. 1 (January 2010): 55–74; T. S Pensabene, *The Rise of the Medical Practitioner in Victoria* (Canberra: Australian National University, 1980), 57–58; E. B. Van Heyningen, "Agents of Empire: The Medical Profession in Cape Colony, 1880–1910," *Medical History* 33 (October 1989): 450–53.

25. In fact, Parliament considered twenty bills—which were either sponsored by individual members or the government—before the medical act was amended in 1886. See Walter Pyke-Lees, *Centenary of the General Medical Council, 1858–1958: The History and Present Work of the Council* (London: GMC, 1959), 7.

26. "General Medical Council on Medical Education and Registration," *British Medical Journal* 2 (July 10, 1869): 38.

27. "General Medical Council on Education and Registration, Session 1867," *British Medical Journal* 1 (June 1, 1867): 640–43.

28. Ibid., 642.

29. "The Week," *Medical Times and Gazette,* February 29, 1868, 234.

30. "General Medical Council," *British Medical Journal* 1 (June 15, 1867): 708.

31. Ibid., 708–9.

32. Ibid., 710.

33. "Medico-Parliamentary: Medical Practitioners (Colonies) Bill," *British Medical Journal* 1 (April 11, 1868): 365.

34. Ronald Hamowy, *Canadian Medicine: A Study in Restricted Entry* (Vancouver, Canada: Fraser Institute, 1984), 68, and D. B. Swinfen, *Imperial Control of Colonial Legislation, 1813–1865: A Study of British Policy towards Colonial Legislative Powers* (Oxford: Clarendon Press, 1970).

35. "The Week," *Medical Times and Gazette*, April 11, 1868, 396. The original London office of the GMC was in Soho Square.

36. "Medico-Parliamentary Medical Practitioners (Colonies) Bill)," *British Medical Journal* 1 (May 2, 1868): 441.

37. Ibid.

38. Shirley Roberts, *Sophia Jex-Blake: A Woman Pioneer in Nineteenth Century Medical Reform* (London: Routledge, 1993), 39, 72.

39. Ibid., 90–124.

40. In 1870 Frances Hogan and Elizabeth Garrett Anderson obtained medical degrees from the University of Paris. Ibid., 99, 154. Compared to Britain, France and Switzerland were more open. But the participation of women in medical education was qualified and limited in numbers. The women admitted were foreign nationals—generally from countries that opposed equal treatment of women, including Austria, Britain, Germany, Russia, and the United States—rather than French and Swiss citizens. Further, a prominent male sponsor on the medical faculty was essential. See Thomas Neville Bonner, *To the Ends of the Earth: Women's Search for Education in Medicine* (Cambridge, MA: Harvard University Press, 1992), 31–56.

41. "General Medical Council: Session 1875," *British Medical Journal* 1 (June 26, 1875): 849.

42. Ibid., 855–56.

43. Roberts, *Sophia Jex-Blake*, 153–54.

44. On women in medicine, see Ann Digby, *The Evolution of British General Practice, 1850–1948*, 154–86. For a discussion of the implication of the LSMW in British rule in India, see Antoinette Burton, "Contesting the Zenana: The Mission to Make 'Lady Doctors for India,' 1874–1885," *Journal of British Studies* 35 (July 1996): 368–97 Female doctors—unlike their male counter-parts—did not pose as disruptive a presence in treating Indian women, particularly in their homes. At the same time, both male and female doctors embraced western medicine as a vehicle for advancing Britain's civilizing mission in colonial India.

45. Bonner, *To the Ends of the Earth*, 133. On the landscape of careers in medicine for women, see Ann Digby, *The Evolution of British General Practice, 1850–1948*, 154–86.

46. On this topic, see Thomas Neville Bonner, *Becoming a Physician: Medical Education in Britain, France, Germany and the United States* (Oxford: Oxford University Press, 1995), and John Harley Warner, *The Therapeutic Perspective: Medical Practice, Knowledge, Identity in America, 1820–1885* (Cambridge, MA: Harvard University Press, 1986).

47. On the combined effect of gender bias and xenophobia in the politics of the professionalization of French medicine in the nineteenth century, see Julie Fette, *Exclusions: Practicing Prejudice in French Law and Medicine, 1920–1945* (Ithaca, NY: Cornell University Press, 2012), 7–14, 19–29. See also Jack D. Ellis, *The Physician-Legislator of France: Medicine and Politics in the Early Third Republic, 1870–1914* (Cambridge: Cambridge University Press, 1990), 145–59.

48. "Abstract I, by the Registrar of the Medical Council, of Documents relating to British and other Foreign Medical Practitioners in France" in "Papers relating to the

Status, under the Medical Act, of Indian, Colonial, and Foreign Practitioners, and of British Practitioners when in France," *Select Committee on the Medical Amendment Act,* XII (1878–1879), appendix, no. 11, 353–54.

49. "Memorandum, by the President of the Medical Council, on the State of the Law and Custom as regards Foreign Medical Practitioners in England, and as to Foreign Medical and Surgical Degrees and Diplomas," ibid., appendix no. 2, 336. This legislative action was anticipated several months earlier by the decision of Public Minister M. Waddington to deny the request of Edward Sparks to practice medicine.

50. Ibid., 353.

51. "Report of the Medical Acts Committee: Territorial Range of Titles to Practice," ibid., 334–35.

52. "General Medical Council: Session 1877," *British Medical Journal* 1 (May 26, 1877): 646.

53. Ibid. Simon acknowledged Corrigan's reasoning: "There was no question as to the goodness of the colonial qualifications; although in some parts of the colonies they might not be so high as those in the United Kingdom."

54. Ibid., 649.

55. Nearly twenty bills to amend the Medical Act were introduced between 1870 and 1881. Pyke-Lees, *Centenary of the General Medical Council, 1858–1958,* 7.

56. "Annus Medicus," *Medical Times and Gazette,* December 28, 1878, 733–35.

57. "The Medical Acts Amendment Bill," *Medical Times and Gazette,* March 1, 1879, 229–30.

58. "General Medical Council," *Medical Times and Gazette,* March 22, 1879, 309. Lord Ripon, a liberal member of the Lords, recommended this provision.

59. Ibid.

60. Ibid., 313.

61. Ibid., 336.

62. Ibid., 335–36.

63. "General Medical Council," *British Medical Journal* 2 (July 26, 1879): 127.

64. Ibid.

65. Ibid.

66. Ibid., 128.

67. Letter from Law Officer to C. L. Peel (Privy Council), July 31, 1879, PC 8/247.

68. See Minutes of Evidence in *Special Report from the Select Committee on Medical Amendment Act,* XII (1878–1879), 218–19.

69. Minutes of Evidence from *Report of the Royal Commission Appointed to Enquire into the Medical Acts* 29 (1882): 61–62.

70. Ibid.

71. Medical Act 1886.

Chapter Two

1. *The Medical Register* (London: General Medical Council, 1914), 1153–54.

2. "British Practitioners Abroad," *British Medical Journal* 2 (August 31, 1901): 567–69. In France a university degree awarded under the same conditions as a French national was required. Those who held British diplomas were exempted from having

to complete the preliminary instruction or to pass an examination in arts and science on the strength of their university degree or evidence having completed equivalent. But this exemption was at the discretion of the minister of public instruction. Even if granted, this degree did not entitle the holder to the right to practice medicine. See also "Special Correspondence: Brussels," *British Medical Journal* 2 (June 9, 1880): 948.

3. "General Medical Council: Summer Session," *British Medical Journal* 1 (June 2, 1890): 1352–53.

4. "The General Medical Council," *British Medical Journal* 2 (December 11, 1897): 1748.

5. Ibid. In contrasting the openness to foreign doctors in Britain, Quain omitted to mention the fact that while foreign doctors could practice without being registered, they were not entitled to the rights of registered doctors, i.e., automatic eligibility for employment in public or imperial service, the right to sue for fees in court, or to sign a death certificate.

6. Ibid.

7. "General Medical Council: Summer Session, 1899," *British Medical Journal* 1 (June 3, 1899): 1369–70.

8. Ibid.

9. Ibid., 1370. The 1886 Act expanded membership on the council to thirty and provided for five members to be directly elected. Long viewed as an institution that represented the interests of the medical establishment—university and nonuniversity licensing bodies—this provision afforded general practitioners with a voice in the regulation of the profession. See Stacey, *Regulating British Medicine*, 20.

10. "General Council of Medical Education and Registration: Summer Session, 1899," *British Medical Journal* 1 (June 17, 1899): 1478.

11. "Reciprocity with Foreign Countries (Stuart Tidey)," *British Medical Journal* 2 (August 12, 1899): 438.

12. "General Medical Council: Summer Session, 1900," *British Medical Journal* 2 (June 2, 1900): 1352.

13. Ibid., 1353–54.

14. Ibid., 1353.

15. Ibid., 1354. Elected to the Council in 1889, MacAlister was later elected president in 1904 and served until 1931.

16. *Medical Register for 1914* (London: Constable & Co, Ltd for GMC, 1914), 1153–54.

17. "The British Practitioner Abroad," *The Lancet* 2 (August, 31, 1912): 662–63.

18. "The Anglo-Japanese Alliance," *British Medical Journal* 1 (January 6, 1906): 39.

19. See John Bowers, *Medical Education in Japan* (New York: Harper & Row, 1965), and John Bowers, *When the Twain Meet: The Rise of Western Medicine in Japan* (Baltimore: Johns Hopkins University Press, 1980).

20. Japanese Minister at Court Hadasu Hayashi, July 21, 1905, to The Marquess of Lansdowne, *GMC Minutes*, appendix 2, part 1.

21. Japanese Minister at Court Hadasu Hayashi, June 23, 1905, to The Marquess of Lansdowne, in "Correspondence in regard to the Proposed Extension of Part II of the Medical act, 1886, to the Empire of Japan," *GMC Minutes*, appendix 2, part 1, 360–61.

22. Ibid.

23. E. Gorst Foreign Office, June 29, 1905, to A. W. Fitzroy Under Secretary of State, Colonial Office, *GMC Minutes*, appendix 2, part 1, 362.

24. Japanese Minister at Court Hadasu Hayashi, July 21, 1905, to the Marquess of Lansdowne, *GMC Minutes*, appendix 2, part 1, 364.

25. GMC Register H. E. Allen, August 3, 1905, to Clerk of the Privy Council, *GMC Minutes*, appendix 2, part 1, 365–66.

26. GMC Acting Registrar A. J. Cockington, March 13, 1916, to Clerk of the Privy Council, *GMC Minutes*, appendix 2, part 1, 131–34.

27. "General Medical Council," *The Lancet* 1 (May 30, 1914): 1574.

28. "Letter from the Members of the Central Sanitary Council of Japan to the Members of the General Medical Council, 1914," in *GMC Minutes*, appendix 10 (Supplementary Correspondence to the Memorandum by the President of the General Council on May 22, 1906, on the Conditions for Medical Qualification in the Japanese Empire), 407–11.

29. Among these included the development and practical application of antitoxin therapy in conferring passive immunity for diphtheria and anthrax as well as the isolation of the plague bacillus during the 1891 outbreak in Hong Kong.

30. "Letter from the Members of the Central Sanitary Council of Japan to the Members of the General Medical Council, 1914," in *GMC Minutes*, appendix 10 (Supplementary Correspondence to the Memorandum by the President of the General Council on May 22, 1906, on the Conditions for Medical Qualification in the Japanese Empire), 407–8.

31. H. W. Just (Colonial Office) March 9, 1916, to the Registrar of the GMC, in *GMC Minutes*, appendix 10 (Supplementary Correspondence to the Memorandum by the President of the General Council on May 22, 1906, on the Conditions for Medical Qualification in the Japanese Empire), 130–31.

32. Ibid., 131.

33. GMC Acting Register A. J. Cockington, March 13, 1916, to The Clerk of the Privy Council, ibid., 131–34.

34. "Regulations of the General Medical Council and Medical Licensing Bodies, Session 1867–1868," *British Medical Journal* 2 (September 14, 1867): 218–34; "General Medical Council on Education and Registration, Session 1869," *British Medical Journal* 2 (July 10, 1869): 38–39; "General Medical Council on Education and Registration," *British Medical Journal* 1 (June 22, 1867): 750–52; "General Medical Council on Education and Registration," *British Medical Journal* 2 (July 24, 1869): 90.

35. A. W. Fitzroy (Privy Council), January 1901 to GMC Registrar H. E. Allen, PC 8/457.

36. "Report of the Education Committee on the Recognition of the Medical Degrees of the University of Malta, June 1901, 13 and 27–28," PC 8/457.

37. "General Council of Medical Education and Registration," *British Medical Journal* 2 (November 30, 1901): 1625.

38. Ronald Hamowy, *Canadian Medicine: A Study in Restricted Entry* (Ottawa: Medical Council of Canada, 1979), 164–262.

39. Ibid., 241. For more on Roddick, see H. E. MacDermot, *Sir Thomas Roddick: His Work in Medicine and Public Life* (Toronto: Macmillan, 1938). Roddick wasted no time in reminding the profession of the advantages of reciprocity when Canada

volunteered medical personnel to serve in the Royal Army Medical Department during the South African War. Lacking registration, they could not practice on British military personnel, only on Canadian troops. See Boyde Beck, "Imperialism and Professionalization: Dominion Registration and Canadian Physicians during the Boer War," *HSTC Bulletin: Journal of the History of Canadian Science, Technology and Medicine/HTSC Bulletin: revue d'historie des science, des techniques et de la medicine au Canada* 8, no. 1 (26) 1984: 3–19.

40. Ibid., 247–54.

41. GMC Registrar H. E. Allen, November 29, 1909, to Clerk of the Privy Council, PC 8/1115.

42. GMC President MacAlister, March 11, 1907, to Lord President of Privy Council, PC 8/1115.

43. Letter from Governor General of Canada (Albert Grey, the Earl of Grey), June 15, 1907, informed the Colonial Secretary (Victor Bruce, 9th Earl of Elgin) that the provincial Medical Board will suggest modifications to the resolution to afford sufficient protection to holders of colonial licenses or diplomas. Letter from Henry E. Allen, May 29, 1908, to Clerk of the Privy Council informing the council that the conditions for reciprocity have been met and therefore such doctors "shall be entitled to be registered in the Colonial List of the Medical Register."

44. GMC Registrar H. E. Allen, November 29, 1909, to Clerk of the Privy Council, PC 8/1115.

45. Medical Board of Quebec Register J. Gauvreau dated January 10, 1910, to GMC Register H. E. Allen, PC 8/1115.

46. Medical Board of Quebec Register J. Gauvreau, February 20, 1910, to GMC Register H. E. Allen, PC 8/1115.

47. GMC Register H. E. Allen, March 17, 1910, to Medical Board of Quebec Register J. Gauvreau, PC 8/1115.

48. GMC President Norman King, May 25, 1911, to Clerk of the Council. PC 8/1115.

49. Prewar income data is incomplete or speculative, but for credible trends see the discussion in Peterson, *Mid-Victorian Medical Profession*, 206–23. Incomes continued to improve after World War I. See Anne Digby and Nick Bosanquet, "Doctors and Patients in an Era of National Health Insurance and Private Practice, 1918–1938," *Economic History Review* 41, no. 1 (1988): 74–94.

50. Anne Digby, *The Evolution of British General Practice, 1850–1948* (Oxford: Oxford University Press, 1999), 67.

51. See Boyde Beck "Imperialism and Professionalization: Dominion Registration and Canadian Physicians during the Boer War," *HSTC Bulletin: Journal of the History of Canadian Science, Technology and Medicine/HTSC Bulletin: revue d'historie des sciences, des techniques et de la medicine au Canada* 8, no. 1 (26) (1984): 3–19.

52. "The War and Medical Reciprocity with Canada," *The Lancet* 1 (April 17, 1915): 833.

53. Robert B. Kerr, *History of the Medical Council of Canada* (Ottawa: The Medical Council of Canada, 1729), 28–29.

54. "Medical Reciprocity with Belgium," *Lancet* 1 (January 16, 1915): 143.

55. "General Council of Medical Education and Registration," *The Lancet* 1 (May 26, 1917): 811.

56. Frederick Taylor, "Memorandum on the Shortage of Medical Students" (August 30, 1917), 1, Ministry of National Service 1/814.

57. Edwin Cornwall, "Memorandum on the Supply of Doctors for the Army" (March 4, 1918), NAT 1/833.

58. "The Man Power Bill," *The Lancet* 1 (April 13 1918): 539.

59. "The General Medical Council of Medical Education and Registration," *The Lancet* 2 (December 1, 1917): 834.

60. Ibid.

Chapter Three

1. "Executive Committee," Minutes of the Medical Council 56 (1919): 6–7.

2. "Special Correspondence: Brussels," *British Medical Journal* 1 (June 19, 1880): 948.

3. "Executive Committee," Minutes of the Medical Council 56 (1919): 7.

4. "The General Medical Council of Medical Education and Registration," *The Lancet* 2 (November 29, 1919): 991.

5. "Executive Committee," Minutes of the General Medical Council 57 (1920): 30.

6. "Registrable Colonial and Foreign Medical Degrees," *The Lancet* 2 (August 27, 1921): 477.

7. H. James Burgwyn, *Italian Foreign Policy in the Interwar Period, 1918–1940* (London: Praeger, 1997).

8. GMC Registrar King, November 30, 1923, to Clerk of the Privy Council, PC 8/1364.

9. H. J. Spon, December 19, 1925, to GMC Registrar Norman King, PC 8/1364.

10. GMC Registrar Norman King, January 1924 to Clerk of the Privy Council, PC 8/1394.

11. GMC Registrar Norman King, February 1, 1924, to Clerk of the Privy Council, PC 8/1394.

12. GMC President MacAlister, February 21, 1925, to Clerk of the Privy Council, PC 8/1394.

13. "The Irish Free State and the Medical and Dentists Act," *The Lancet* 1 (April 11, 1925): 776.

14. Ibid. John F. Fleetwood, *The History of Medicine in Ireland* (Dublin: Skelling Press, 1983), 272–79. In a discussion of the reform of medical education during the interwar period, Greta Jones underscores the importance of national politics in medicine. See Greta Jones, "The Rockefeller Foundation and Medical Education in Ireland in the 1920s," *Irish Historical Studies* 30, no. 120 (November 1997): 564–80.

15. The agreement preserved the role of university and nonuniversity licensing bodies to nominate council representatives while delegating to the governor of Northern Ireland the authority to recommend to Her Majesty in Council a member to represent Northern Ireland. *Agreement between Great Britain, the Irish Free State and Northern Ireland as to the Registration and Control of Medical Practitioners*, schedule part 1, 17 and 18 Geo. 5 Medical and Dentists Amendment Act, 1927, MH 153/709.

16. "The Irish Free State and the Medical and Dentists Act," *The Lancet* 1 (April 11, 1925): 776.

17. "Confidential Memorandum Council President Sir Donald MacAlister in Letter from Colin Smith (Privy Council), March 14, 1928, to J. E. Stephenson (Dominions Office), PC 8/1125. On the occupational mobility of Irish medical graduates, see Greta Jones, "'Strike out Boldly for the Prizes that are Available to You': Medical Emigration from Ireland, 1870–1905," *Medical History* 54, no. 1 (January 2010): 55–74.

18. "Memorandum on difficulties which have arisen under the present system of arrangement for reciprocal acceptance of medical qualifications between the United Kingdom and the Dominions," 6, PC 8/1125.

19. Saskatchewan College of Physicians and Surgeon Registrar A. MacG. Young, February 28, 1924, to GMC Registrar Norman King, PC 8/1078.

20. Saskatchewan College of Physicians and Surgeon Registrar A. MacG. Young, August 15, 1924, to GMC Registrar Normal King, PC 8/1078.

21. GMC Registrar Norman King, September 2, 1924, to Saskatchewan College of Physicians and Surgeon Register A. MacG. Young, PC 8/1078.

22. Quoted in H. Wilberforce Aikins, Registrar, The College of Physicians and Surgeons of Ontario, September 20, 1927, to GMC Registrar Norman King, PC 8/1112.

23. Ibid. Regarding Italy, Aikins wrote, "Your Council through official channels, without asking our College, as one of the parties to the pact between your Council and our College, to agree to the same, entered into arrangement between Great Britain and the Kingdom of Italy, to effect reciprocity between it and Great Britain, granting duly certificated Italian doctors in the British *Register*, and through its certificate admission to the Province of Ontario."

24. GMC Registrar Norman King to H. Wilberforce Aikins, October 27, 1927, PC 8/1112.

25. Ibid.

26. GMC Registrar Norman King, August 11, 1927, to Sir Lindo Ferguson, Chairman of the New Zealand Medical Council, PC 8/1112.

27. Ibid.

28. Ibid.

29. Note to Clerk of the Privy Council Sir Maurice Hankey, February 23, 1929, PC 8/1158.

30. "Medical Act 1886: Opinion of the Law Officers of the Crown, February 4, 1929," PC 8/1158.

31. Ibid.

32. Dominions Office Memorandum, May 1929, enclosure in H. F. Batterbee (Dominions Office), May 16, 1929, to W. E. Beckett (Foreign Office), PC 8/1158, 2.

33. Ibid., 3.

34. Memorandum to Sir Maurice Hankey, February, 23, 1929, PC 8/1158.

35. Maurice Olivier, ed., *The Colonial and Imperial Conferences, 1887–1939*, pt. 2, vol. 3 (Ottawa: Edmond Cloutier, 1954), 150–57. W. E. Beckett (Foreign Office), December 10, 1929, to Colin Smith, Privy Council, PC 8/1158.

36. GMC Registrar Norman King, August 11, 1927, to Chair, New Zealand Medical Council, PC 8/1112.

37. See chapter 1 above.

38. Section 13, part 2, Medical Act 1886, ch. 48, 49 and 50 Vict.

39. India Office, November 5, 1918, Executive Committee (November 25, 1918), Minutes of the Medical Council 55 (1918): 147.

40. Ibid., 148.

41. Ibid., 149.

42. Ibid.

43. "President's Address (November 21, 1921)," Minutes of the General Council 58 (1921): 32.

44. (Executive Committee) Minutes of the General Council 58 (1921): 129.

45. "Annotations: Indian Universities and Midwifery," *Lancet* 1 (January 14, 1922): 87.

46. *Minutes of Medical Council* 59 (1922): 155–69. He planned to visit Madras but could not due to the physical strains of the heat (167).

47. Ibid., 168.

48. Ibid., 158.

49. Ibid., 159.

50. Ibid., 161–67. Common among upper-class Muslims and upper-caste Hindu communities, purdah refers to the organization of domestic spaces that secluded women from public view or separated the sexes. It too extended to practices such as covering the body to minimize revealing the skin or body shape.

51. Ibid., 167.

52. Ibid., 168.

53. Minutes of the Medical Council 60 (1923): 63.

54. Ibid., 62.

55. "The Medical Education Crisis in Bengal," *Indian Medical Gazette,* June 1915, 274.

56. Ibid., 61–62.

57. Minutes of the Medical Council 64 (1927): 391–416.

58. Ibid., 394–95.

59. Ibid., 395.

60. Ibid., 398.

61. Ibid., 416.

62. Ibid.

63. Roger Jeffrey, "Recognizing India's Doctors," *Modern Asian Studies* 13, no. 2 (1979): 307.

64. "The Indian Medical Council: A Retrospect," *Journal of the Indian Medical Association* 8, no. 2 (November 1938): 95–96.

65. "The Indian Medical Council," *Journal of the Indian Medical Association,* 3, no. 12 (August 1934): 530–32.

Chapter Four

1. Kenneth Collins, *Go and Learn: The International Story of Jews and Medicine in Scotland* (Aberdeen: Aberdeen University Press, 1988), and Decker, "Divisions and Diversity," 850–73. In a study, Paul Weindling qualifies the scope of anti-Semitism as a dominant factor in the participation of Jewish refugees in medicine. See his "Medical

Refugees and the Modernisation of British Medicine," *Social History of Medicine* 22, no. 3 (2009): 489–511.

2. John M. Efron, *Medicine and the German Jews: A History* (New Haven, CT: Yale University Press, 2001), 234–36.

3. Ibid., 238–40.

4. Ibid., 263–64.

5. Thomas Neville Bonner, *Becoming a Physician: Medical Education in Britain, France, Germany, and the United States, 1750–1945* (Oxford: Oxford University Press, 1995), 315–16.

6. Collins, *Go and Learn*, 83, 8, 89, 98–130.

7. Todd M. Endelman, *The Jews of Britain, 1656 to 2000* (Berkeley: University of California Press, 2002), 165.

8. Louise London, *Whitehall and the Jews: British Immigration Policy, Jewish Refugees and the Holocaust* (Cambridge: Cambridge University Press, 2000), 16–18, 27.

9. Endelman, *The Jews of Britain*, 211–15.

10. London, *Whitehall and the Jews*, 47–52.

11. Collins, *Go and Learn*, 135.

12. Ibid., 133–39. Still, the Conjoint Board agreed to decrease the number of admissions to one from six per year. See Karola Decker, "Divisions and Diversity: The Complexities of Medical Refuge in Britain, 1933–1948," *Bulletin of the History of Medicine* 77 (2003): 852.

13. E. C. E. Leadbitter (Privy Council), July 24, 1935, to Lord President, PC 8/1294.

14. Karola Decker, "Divisions and Diversity: The Complexities of Medical Refuge in Britain, 1933–1948," *Bulletin of the History of Medicine* 77 (2003): 852–54.

15. Ibid. For its part, the role of the GMC was prescribed by statute. Even though the nonuniversity licensing bodies had representatives on the council, the GMC itself lacked independent authority over requalification. This was a right that medical bodies retained as part of the compromise that had led to the creation of the GMC in 1858.

16. GMC Registrar Michael Helestine, July 31, 1933, to Colin Smith (Privy Council), PC 8/1364.

17. Ibid.

18. Renzo Del Felice, *The Jews in Fascist Italy* (New York: Engima Books, 2001).

19. GMC Registrar Michael Helestine, December 10, 1935, to E. C. E. Leadbitter (Privy Council), PC 8/1364.

20. GMC Registrar Michael Helestine, April 26, 1935, to E. C. E. Leadbitter (Privy Council), PC 8/1364.

21. Executive Committee, Minutes of the General Medical Council, November 21, 1938, PC 8/1364.

22. GMC Registrar Michael Helestine, December 5, 1938, to Clerk of the Privy Council, PC 8/1364.

23. John Samos, legal advisor to the Foreign Office, March 24, 1939, to GMC Registrar Michael Helestine, PC 8/1364.

24. "Victoria's Restrictions on Alien Doctors," London *Times*, June 7, 1939, 15, col. C.

25. "Foreign Doctors in N.S.W.: Severe Restrictions," London *Times*, August 9, 1939, 11, col. F.

26. John Weaver, "'A Glut on the Market': Medical Practice Laws and Treatment of Refugee Doctors in Australia and New Zealand, 1933–1942" (unpublished manuscript), 18–21.

27. "G.M.C.: Winter Session," *British Medical Journal* 2 (November 26, 1938): 336.

28. Ibid.

29. "G.M.C.: Summer Session," *British Medical Journal Supplement* 1 (May 27, 1939): 299.

30. "Victoria's Restrictions on Alien Doctors," London *Times*, June 7, 1939, 15.

31. Karola, "Medical Refuge in Britain, 1933–1948," 864.

32. "Canadian and American Doctors for the E.M.S.," *Lancet* 2 (September 28, 1940): 398.

33. There were two routes to the register for full registration or unrestricted rights to practice: the possession of medical qualifications recognized by the GMC awarded in a reciprocating country and obtaining a primary qualification in the United Kingdom through requalification.

34. Letter from Michiels van Verduynen, Netherlands Legation, June 7, 1940, to Viscount Halifax, PO 8/1395.

35. Memorandum on the Grant of Facilities to Practice in the United Kingdom to Netherland Doctors and Dentists, 2, PO 8/1395. Helestine doubted that even if such doctors received a work permit, they would be permitted to prescribe medication.

36. Ibid.

37. "Circular 2264: Temporary Registration and Employment of Overseas Medical Practitioners," January 15, 1941, MH 76/334.

38. "Temporary Registration of Overseas Medical Practitioners: Memorandum by the Lord President of the Council, Home Secretary, the Minister of Health, and the Secretary of State for Scotland, August 22, 1941, CAB 75/12/52.

39. Notes on Meeting with the GMC President, July 31, 1941, MH 76/334.

40. GMC Registrar Michael Helestine, September 13, 1940, to W. E. Beckett, MH 76/334.

41. "Observations on Draft of Medical Register on Temporary Registration Order, No. 2, 1941," MH 76/334.

42. "Employment of Alien Doctors and Nurses in Hospitals," *British Medical Journal* 2 (November 9, 1940): 653.

43. R. A. Gallop (Foreign Office), May 3, 1941, to A. W. Neville, MH 76/334.

44. J. N. Beckett (Ministry of Health), May 21, 1941, to R. A. Gallop (Foreign Office), MH 76/334.

45. A. W. G. Randall (Foreign Office), May 21, 1941, MH /76/334.

46. Ibid.

47. "General Medical Council: Observations on Draft (July 7, 1941) of Medical Register (Temporary Registration) Order No. 2, 1941," 1, MH 74/334.

48. Ibid., 2.

49. Ibid.

50. Ibid., 3–4.

51. Ibid., 4–5.

52. A. W. Randall, July 31, 1941, to Chief Medical Office and Deputy Secretary, MH 76/334.

53. Draft Order in Council Substituting a New Regulation for Regulation 32B of the Defense (General) Regulation, 1939, CAB 75/12/52.

54. Decker, "Divisions and Diversity," 869–72.

55. Foreign doctors who had arrived in Britain after the end of temporary registration were also eligible to apply.

56. General Medical Council, Memorandum on the Registration of Commonwealth and Foreign Doctors, October 1967, 10, MH 153/548.

57. Ibid.

58. "End of the Temporary Register," *The Lancet* 2 (August 9, 1947): 225.

59. General Medical Council, Memorandum on the Registration of Commonwealth and Foreign Doctors, October 1967, 10, MH 153/548.

Chapter Five

1. On the history of naturalization, see M. Page Baldwin, "Subject to Empire: Married Women and the British Nationality and Status of Aliens Act," *Journal of British Studies* 40 (October 2001): 522–56.

2. Mary Ann Elston, "Medicine: Half Our Future Doctors," in *Careers of Professional Women,* ed. Rosalie Silverstone and Audrey War (London: Croom Helm, 1980): 99–134.

3. *Report of the Committee to Consider the Future Numbers of Medical Practitioners and the Appropriate Intake of Medical Students* (London: H.M. Stationary Office, 1957). Henry Willink was a former conservative minister of health in the wartime coalition government (1943–45).

4. Ibid., 2–3.

5. Ibid., 32.

6. Ibid.

7. Ibid., 33–34.

8. Ibid., 26, 29.

9. Ibid., 33. The yield assumed a 6 percent attrition of medical students.

10. Francois Lafitte and John Squire, "Special Articles: Second Thoughts on the Willink Report," *The Lancet* 2 (September 3, 1960): 538–41. See also "Supply of Doctors," London *Times,* November 22, 1957, 13. For a discussion of the deficiencies in postwar planning, see Stephen Birch, Alan Maynard, and Arthur Walker, "Doctor Manpower Planning in the United Kingdom: Problems Arising from Myopia," Discussion Paper 18, Center for Health Economics, University of York, August 1986.

11. See "Shortage of Doctors to be Remedied," London *Times,* November 30, 1961, 18, and Anthony Barber MP, cited in *Hansard* 1963: col. 686.

12. This overview of registration trends is based on data provided in the General Medical Council, Memorandum on the Registration of Commonwealth and Foreign Doctors, October 1967, sections 1–3, appendix 1, MH 153/548.

13. Beginning in 1953, all candidates for full registration were required to complete a preregistration year of training in an approved hospital. This requirement

applied to overseas doctors from reciprocating countries unless they could provide evidence of equivalent training.

14. It is important to note that these totals do not necessarily reflect unique applications because doctors had to reapply either when they changed positions or the period of temporary registration expired.

15. "Doctors from Everywhere: London as a Postgraduate Medical Centre," London *Times*, October 31, 1956, 9.

16. "General Medical Council," *The Lancet* 1 (June 1, 1957): 1142.

17. Ibid., *Lancet* 2 (December 4, 1965): 1179.

18. Ibid. Lord Birkenhead was also a member of the Willink Commission.

19. "General Medical Council," *The Lancet* 2 (December 4, 1965): 1179.

20. "Memorandum by the General Medical Council on Registration Fees," *British Medical Journal* 1 (May 7, 1966): 1164.

21. This is based on an analysis of the Expenditure and Income statements of the GMC for the years 1965–69.

22. "Memorandum by the General Medical Council on Registration Fees," *British Medical Journal* 1 (May 7, 1966): 1164. It is noteworthy that doctors registered in Ireland—a republic with its own registration system—did not have to pay 6 pounds for provisional registration whereas doctors from the Commonwealth did. Irish doctors were required to pay 12 pounds for full registration (like British doctors), but Commonwealth doctors as well as foreign-trained doctors, who requalified, were charged 16 pounds. See "General Medical Council," *The Lancet* 1 (June 1, 1963): 1203.

23. As early as 1962, the GMC relied on these fees to make up deficit in the operating budget as costs rose and other sources of revenue remained flat. "Memorandum by the General Medical Council on Registration Fees," *British Medical Journal* 1 (May 7, 1966): 1164.

24. Ibid.

25. For a discussion of this relation, see Douglas M. Haynes, "Social Status and Imperial Service: Tropical Medicine and the British Medical Profession in the Nineteenth Century," in *Warm Climates and Western Medicine: The Emergence of Tropical Medicine, 1500–1900*, ed. David Arnold (Amsterdam: Rodopi, 1996), 208–20.

26. Anne Digby and Nick Bosanquet, "Doctors and Patients in an Era of National Health Insurance and Private Practice, 1913–1938," *Economic History Review* 41, no. 1 (1988): 80–86, and on the process of Indianization, see Roger Jeffery, "Recognizing India's Doctors: The Institutionalization of Medical Dependency, 1918–1939," *Modern Asian Studies* 13, no. 2 (1979): 301–26.

27. Brian Abel-Smith and Kathleen Gales, *British Doctors at Home and Abroad* (Welwyn, UK: Published for the Social Administration Research Trust by Codicote Press, 1964), 56.

28. See *Royal Commission Report on Medical Education, 1965–1968* (London: Her Majesty's Stationary Office, 1968), 27–43. This report is also known as the Todd Report.

29. The Nuffield Provincial Hospitals Trust, *Seventh Report, Postgraduate Medical Education: A Record of Progress of Schemes and Descriptions of New Projects* (Nuffield, UK: The Nuffield Provincial Hospitals Trust, 1964). For an overview of British training in

medical specializations, see George Weisz, *Divide and Conquer: A Comparative History of Medical Specialization* (Oxford: Oxford University Press, 2006), 164–87.

30. *Report of the Joint Working Party on the Medical Staffing Structure in the Hospital Service* (London: Her Majesty's Stationary Office, 1961). This report is also known as the Platt Report.

31. Ibid., 28–32.

32. Ibid., 32.

33. "Questions in the Commons: Contracting Out of the Service and Doctors from Overseas," *British Medical Journal* 2, no. 1720 (December 23, 1961): 1720.

34. John Seale, "Medical Emigration from Britain, 1930–1961," *British Medical Journal* 1, no. 5280 (March 17, 1962): 782–86.

35. Ibid., 785.

36. Mary Ann Elton, "Medicine," in *Careers of Professional Women*: 105–8.

37. "Women Medical Graduates," *Lancet* 1 (June 20, 1964): 1387.

38. "Annual Conference of Local Medical Committees," *British Medical Journal* 1 (June 16, 1962): 267–68. As a conservative backbencher in Parliament, Powell gained notoriety for being a staunch opponent of immigration to Britain from "new" Commonwealth countries in Africa and the Caribbean as well as India and Pakistan.

39. Ibid., 268.

40. Ibid., 269.

41. "Medical Notes in Parliament: N.H.S. Staffing in the Context of a Strained Economy," *British Medical Journal* 1 (April 7, 1962): 1018.

42. Ibid., 1019.

43. "Emigration of British Doctors," *British Medical Journal* 1 (April 14, 1964): 1074–75.

44. Ibid., 2 (July 4, 1964): 2.

45. Ibid.

46. General Medical Council, Memorandum on the Registration of Commonwealth and Foreign Doctors, October 1967, section 3 of appendix 3, 5, MH 153/548.

47. Ibid., appendix 2, section 2, 1.

48. Ibid., appendix 3, section 3, 5.

49. "Marriage and the G.M.C. [Annotations]," *The Lancet* 2 (August 19, 1967): 408.

50. "The Temporary Register," *The Lancet* 2 (December 2, 1967): 1192.

51. Ibid.

52. "Temporary Registration and Re-qualification," *The Lancet* 2 (December 2, 1967): 1200.

53. Ibid.

54. Ibid., 1201.

55. "The Temporary Register," *The Lancet* 2 (December 9, 1967): 1252.

56. "Postgraduate Training Posts for Overseas Doctors," *British Medical Journal* 1 (February 26, 1966): 545.

57. Ibid.

58. "Postgraduate Training Posts for Overseas Doctors," *British Medical Journal* 1 (April 2, 1966): 863.

59. Ibid. (March 19, 1966), 740.

60. "BMA Seeks Talks on Registration," London *Times*, August 22, 1967, 3.

61. "The Temporary Register," *The Lancet* 2 (December 2, 1967): 1192.

62. Sir Cyril Black, House of Commons Debate, *Hansard*, May 15, 1968, vol. 764, cc1361.

63. "Examinations in English for Overseas Graduates (L.R.M. Kamal)," *British Medical Journal* 1, no. 5489 (March 19, 1966): 740.

64. P. J. Cashman to Walker Pyke-Lees, August 23, 1967, MH 153/548.

65. General Medical Council, Memorandum on the Registration of Commonwealth and Foreign Doctors, October 1967, MH 153/548.

66. Ibid., 1.

67. Ibid., 4.

68. Ibid., 5.

69. Ibid., 6.

70. Ibid.

71. "Summary, and Suggestions in Connection with Any Amending Legislation," in General Medical Council, Memorandum on the Registration of Commonwealth and Foreign Doctors, October 1967, 14, MH 153/548.

72. Ibid.

73. Ibid., 15.

74. Ibid., 16.

75. Ibid., 17.

76. "General Medical Council," *British Medical Journal Supplement* 4 (December 7, 1968): 53.

77. "Overseas Doctors," *British Medical Journal* 1 (March 22, 1969): 730.

78. Rosemary Stevens and Joan Vermeulen, *Foreign Trained Physicians and American Medicine*, DHEW Publication No. (NIH) 73-325, June 1972: 26–35. For a case study of the pre-ECFMG examination, see Greta Jones, "The Rockefeller Foundation and Medical Education in Ireland in the 1920s," *Irish Historical Studies* 30, no. 120 (November 1997): 564–80.

Chapter Six

1. Kathleen Paul, *Whitewashing Britain: Race and Citizenship in the Postwar Era* (Ithaca, NY: Cornell University Press, 1997), 166–67.

2. This remained the case after the implementation of provisional registration in 1953 and after the council increased registration fees in 1965.

3. "Annual Registration Fees," *British Medical Journal* 1 (May 7, 1966): 1130–31.

4. "Memorandum by the General Medical Council," *British Medical Journal* 1 (May 7, 1966): 1164.

5. Ibid.

6. "Annual Report of Council," *British Medical Journal Supplement* 1 (May 14, 1966): 187.

7. "Annual Registration Fees," *British Medical Journal* 1 (May 7, 1966): 1130–31.

8. Cited in Christopher Kyriakides and Satnam Virdee, "Migrant Labour. Racism and the British National Health Service," *Ethnicity and Health* 8, no. 4 (November 2003): 289.

9. "Overseas Graduates," *British Medical Journal* 1 (March 10, 1962): 713.

10. A. G. W. Whitfield and J. McCall, "Commonwealth Schools," *The Lancet* 1 (June 15, 1963): 1318–19.

11. "Report on Attachment Scheme for Overseas Doctors," MH 149/1003, 1–3.

12. "Overseas Doctors: Memorandum by the Department of Health and Social Security, the Scottish Home and Health Department and the Welsh Office," MH 149/1076, 3.

13. "Annual Clinical Meeting," *British Medical Journal* 1 (March 22, 1969): 106–7.

14. "Doctors from Overseas," *British Medical Journal* 1 (March 22, 1969): 730.

15. "Testing by the General Medical Council, Appendix I," 1–4, MH149/1004.

16. Ibid.

17. Ibid., 2.

18. French President De Gaulle vetoed previous applications in 1963 and 1967.

19. Ibid., 3.

20. Ibid., 2.

21. Richard Crossman, *The Diaries of a Cabinet Minister*, vol. 3, *Secretary of State for Social Service, 1968–1970* (London: Hamish Hamilton and Jonathan Cape, 1977), 400, 412.

22. Ibid.

23. "Meeting with BMA on Overseas Doctors, 20th March 1969: Brief for Secretary of State, Speaking Notes," 1, MH 149/1004.

24. Ibid., 2.

25. Ibid.

26. Ibid.

27. "Note on Meeting with the BMA about overseas doctors, held on 20 March 1969," MH 149/1004.

28. "Improving the Attachment Scheme," *The Lancet* 1 (June 28, 1969): 1325.

29. GeneralMe.dical Council, Interim Report of the Special Committee on the Registration of Overseas Doctors, February 1972, 1, MH 149/1827.

30. Ibid.

31. Ibid., 6.

32. The report continued in a similar vein: "There was a similar feeling that a small proportion of overseas doctors may find some difficulty in adapting themselves to the habits and attitudes of patient care which have become established in this country." Ibid., 6.

33. Ibid., 7.

34. "The need for and value of reciprocity in the arrangements for the registration of overseas doctors (Part III)." Ibid., 7.

35. Ibid.

36. Ibid.

37. Ibid., 5.

38. Ibid.

39. "The relative merits of systems based primarily on recognition of qualifications and those based primarily on an examination or assessment of the individual: possible combination of the two systems (Part I)." Ibid., 2–4.

40. General Medical Council, Interim Report of the Special Committee on the Registration of Overseas Doctors, 7–8.

41. "Problems arising from language difficulties or from unfamiliarity with the circumstances of medical practice in this country. The feasibility of making increased use of the Clinical Attachment Scheme within the National Health Service to assess the professional and linguistic competence of applicants for registration (Part II)." Ibid., 5–6.

42. Ibid., 8–12.

43. R. Cattran on "Registration of Overseas Doctors: GMC's Proposed New Arrangements," December 20, 1971, MH 149/1827.

44. "Registration of Overseas Doctors: Memorandum of Evidence by Department of Health and Social Security," MH 147/1827.

45. "British Medical Association: Comments on the Interim Report of the Special Committee on the Registration of Overseas Doctors (July 27, 1972)," 1–5, MH147/1827.

46. There were three postgraduate councils: England and Wales, Scotland, and Northern Ireland. See reference in "British Medical Association Working Party on the Functions of the General Medical Council," *British Medical Journal Supplement* 4 (November 11, 1972): 34.

47. "Comments on the Interim Report of Special Committee of the General Medical Council Concerning the Registration of Overseas Doctors," by the Scottish Council for Postgraduate Medical Education, MH147/1827, 2–3.

48. Ibid.

49. Ibid., 2

50. "British Medical Association Special Representative Meeting," *British Medical Journal Supplement* 1 (February 21, 1970): 51–62. This was the day before notifying the Privy Council.

51. Ibid., 51.

52. Ibid., 53, 57, 59.

53. Ibid., 52–53, 55–56.

54. Ibid., 60.

55. Ibid., 61.

56. G. E. Godber to Alfred Bavin, February 24, 1970, MH 153/466.

57. Ibid.

58. P. Brenner to Alfred Bavin, February 25, 1970, MH 153/466.

59. Ibid.

60. "Note on Meeting to Discuss the Constitution of the GMC," by Dr. Elizabeth Shore, March 11, 1970, 1–3, MH 153/466. See also Stacey, *Regulating British Medicine,* 37.

61. "Note on Meeting to Discuss the Constitution of the GMC," by Dr. Elizabeth Shore, March 11, 1970, 1, MH 153/466.

62. Ibid., 1–2. Cohen's view about the age difference was not isolated. See Stacey, *Regulating British Medicine,* 74.

63. Ibid., 3.

64. Ibid.

65. "Composition of the General Medical Council Report of Working Party," *British Medical Journal Supplement* 1 (March 6, 1971): 55–62.

66. Ibid., 58.

67. Ibid.

68. Ibid., 60.

69. "General Medical Council," *British Medical Journal Supplement* 4 (December 11, 1971): 61.

70. Stacey, *Regulating British Medicine,* 41.

71. "General Medical Council," *British Medical Journal Supplement* 4 (December 11, 1971): 72.

72. Ibid.

73. "Proceedings of the Council," *British Medical Journal Supplement* 4 (December 11, 1971): 61–62.

74. Ibid., 4 (March 11, 1972): 62.

75. Ibid.

76. "Annual Representative Meeting," *British Medical Journal Supplement* 3 (July 29, 1972): 89–93.

77. Ibid., 93.

78. Ibid., 91.

79. "British Medical Association and General Medical Council: Working Group on the Functions of the General Medical Council," *British Medical Journal Supplement* 4 (November 11, 1972): 33.

80. Ibid., 34.

81. Ibid., 35.

82. Stacey, *Regulating British Medicine,* 29–41.

83. Martin Draper (GMC) to Robert Cattran (DHSS), October 17, 1972, MH 149/1827.

Chapter Seven

1. Paul, *Whitewashing Britain,* 179–84.

2. Zig Layton-Henry, "Immigration and the Heath Government," in *The Heath Government,* ed. Stuart Ball and Anthony Seldon (Harlow, UK: Addison Wesley Longman Group, 1996), 227.

3. H. Yellowlees, CMO, to Sir John Richardson, President, GMC, July 27, 1972, MH153/770.

4. The medical schools affected in Pakistan included University of Decca (Dacca Medical College); University of Karachi (Dow Medical College); University of Peshawar (Khyber Medical College); University of Punjab (King Edward College, Lahore); Fatima Jinnah Medical College for Women; Nishtar Medical College, Multan; and University of Sind (Liaquat Medical College, Hyderabad). *Annual Report of the General Medical Council* (1972), Report of Overseas Committee (appendix 16), 294.

5. The 1962 Medical Practitioners (Republic of South Africa Order) replaced the original 1921 order when it was a member of the Commonwealth. Department of Health and Social Security Application to the Law Officers of the Crown Order-In-Council Dated 8 May 1896 and Medical Act 1956, MH 153/700.

6. Department of Health and Society Security Application to Law Officers of the Crown, Order-in-Council Dated 8 May 1892 and Medical Act 1956, MH 153/770.

7. Ibid.

8. CMO H. Yellowlees to GMC President Sir John Richardson, July 27, 1972, MH153/770.

9. "Special Committee on the Registration of Overseas Doctors (November 1973), Appendix X," *Annual Report of the General Medical Council for 1973* (1974), 255.

10. Ibid., 197–98.

11. Overseas Committee, "Review of Overseas Qualifications Recognized for Full Registration (May 1973)," appendix 9, *Annual Report of the General Medical Council for 1973* (1974), 250–51.

12. Ibid., 250.

13. Ibid., 251.

14. Ibid.

15. Cohen doubted that exporting countries like India would host such a test because the USFMG test facilitated the emigration of its doctors.

16. Martin Draper, GMC Register, to DHSS Assistant Secretary R. Cattran, October 17, 1972, MH 149/1827.

17. Memo R. Cattran to Dr Shore and Dr Cohen re: Interim Report, June 19, 1972, MH 149/1827.

18. Memo P. Brenner to Dr. Cohen on Cattran, June 27, 1972, MH 149/1827.

19. Memo Benner to Robertson, July 14, 1972, MH 149/1827.

20. Ibid.

21. Ibid.

22. Memo from R. Cattran on Draper to Brenner, Dr. Reid, and Dr. Shore, October 10, 1972, MH 149/1827.

23. Ibid.

24. Memo Robertson to Nodder, December 8, 1972, MH 149/1827.

25. Note on a Meeting held on July 24, 1973, between representatives of the Examining Board in Scotland, the Society of Apothecaries of London, and the General Medical Council, MH 149/1828.

26. Note on a Meeting held on March 1, 1973, between representatives of the Examining Board in Scotland, the Society of Apothecaries of London, and the General Medical Council, MH 149/1828.

27. Ibid.

28. Note on a Meeting held on June 27, 1973, between representatives of the Examining Board in Scotland, the Society of Apothecaries of London, and the General Medical Council, MH 149/1828. At the same, Hunt added that "clinical proficiency should be tested at a clinical interview (without patients) by two pairs of Assessors (one in general medicine and a specialty, the other in surgery and obstetrics)."

29. "Report of the Working Party to the Royal Colleges and Society of Apothecary via the Committee of Management of the three Non-university Licensing Bodies Report (March 1974)," Minutes of the Royal College of Physician Comitia.

30. Ibid. The report proposed that the current working party "be appointed for an initial period of one year (renewable) and that a Report be submitted to the Colleges and Society via the Licensing Bodies in April 1975."

31. J. G. Hall to Dr. Elizabeth Shore, March 8, 1974, MH149/1829.

32. "Revision of the Attachment for Overseas Doctors," MH149/1828.

33. Of the 3,602, J. G. Hall assumed that the majority of these applicants ultimately did not travel to Britain after all. J. G. Hall to Cattran and Wintergill, March 8, 1974, MH149/1829.

34. DHSS provided for four exemption categories for overseas-trained doctors who (1) were sponsored under a technical training or scholarship program; (2) accepted a prearranged appointment at the grade of registrar or higher; (3) completed a three-month or more postgraduate certificate course at a university or an institution of equivalent status; and (4) possessed a testimonial from a refugee familiar to the hospital board testifying to the candidate's suitability for an appointment and facility with the English language. "Revision of the Attachment Scheme for Overseas Doctors," MH149/1828.

35. Note of Meeting on Monday, March 1, 1974, to Discuss GMC Proposals for Tests for Overseas Doctors, MH149/1829; Internal Paper: GMC Proposals for Tests for Overseas Doctors, December 10, 1974, MH 149/1833; and Joan Firth to Nodder, January 15, 1975, MH 149/1833. In the final arrangements, the GMC determined exemption to testing while hospital authorities would be responsible for scheduling test times and venues for clinical attachment applicants.

36. GMC Proposals for Tests of Overseas Doctors: Informal Meeting with the Home Office on November 15, 1974, MH149/1833.

37. "Note on a Meeting 27 June 1973 Between Representatives of the Examining Board in England, of the Board of Management of the Scottish Triple Qualification, and of the Society of Apothecaries of London" and "Note of a Meeting 14 September 1973 Between Representatives from the DHSS and the GMC," MH149/1828.

38. Joan Firth to Scales, January 21, 1975, MH 149/1833.

39. "Draft Letter to Regional and Area Health Authorities," MH 149/1833.

40. Ibid.

41. "Joint Consultants Committee: Attachment Scheme for Overseas Doctors," *British Medical Journal* 3, no. 5926 (August 3, 1974): 359.

42. "Joint Consultants Committee," *British Medical Journal* 1, no. 5953 (February 8, 1975): 349.

43. "Overseas Doctors: Note for Ministers," by Joan Firth, November 19, 1974, MH 149/1833.

44. "Joint Consultants Committee," *British Medical Journal* 1, no. 5953 (February 8, 1975): 349.

45. Ibid., 350.

46. Dr. Gullick (JCC) to Martin Draper (GMC), March 5, 1975, MH 149/ 1834.

47. Royal College of Physicians Comitia (Minutes), Annals (vol. 77), 13–19.

48. Ibid., 16.

49. Ibid., 21.

50. Ibid.

51. Ibid., 23.

52. Ibid., 29.

53. Ibid., 31.

54. Ibid., 33.

55. Ibid.

56. Dr. Gullick (JCC) to Martin Draper (GMC), March 5, 1975, MH 149/ 1834.

57. Martin Draper to Joan Firth, March 3, 1975, MH 149/1834.

58. Joan Firth to Dr. Wintersgill, March 5, 1975, NH 149/1834.

Chapter Eight

1. Martin Draper (GMC) to N. E. Leigh (Clerk of the Privy Council Office), December 6, 1974, MH149/1829.

2. Martin Draper to R. Cattran, October 17, 1972, MH 149/1827.

3. Martin R. Draper to Lake, February 21, 1975, MH 149/773.

4. Ibid.

5. "Medical Manpower: Appreciation of the Effect of Withdrawal of Recognition from Indian Medical Schools," MH 149/1829, 1–3.

6. Ibid., 2–3.

7. Ibid., 2.

8. Ibid., 3.

9. W. F. X White to George Chalmers, February 25, 1975, CO MH 153/773.

10. Ibid.

11. N. E. Leigh (Privy Council) to Martin Draper (GMC), May 8, 1975, MH 153/773.

12. Ibid.

13. Draft Submission, No Date, MH149/1834.

14. Ibid. In a letter to Joan Firth, Nigel Sharp thought so, too: "The Merrison Report may help towards the acceptance of the GMC's prospective decision on India as reasonable though I imagine that the Government will not wish to state its views on individual recommendations including those on overseas doctors at this stage." N. E. Sharp to Joan Firth (DHSS), April 8, 1975, MH 153/773.

15. *Report of the Committee of Inquiry into the Regulation of the Medical Profession* (London: Her Majesty's Stationary Office, 1974–75), ii–iii.

16. Ibid., 157–60.

17. Ibid., 53.

18. Ibid., 55.

19. Ibid., 58–59.

20. Weisz, *Divide and Conquer*, 164–87.

21. *Report of the Committee of Inquiry into the Regulation of the Medical Profession*, 58–59.

22. Ibid. This view of overseas health professionals extended to nurses as well. See The Royal College of Nursing and National Council of Nurses of the United Kingdom, *RCN Evidence to the Committee on Nursing* (London, 1971), paras. 62 and 30.

23. On Britain's reliance on overseas nurses of color, see Emma L. Jones and Stephanie J. Snow, *"Against the Odds": Black and Minority Ethnic Clinicians and Manchester, 1948–2009* (Manchester, UK: Manchester NHS Primary Care Trust, 2010), 8–10, 50–69.

24. Ibid., 61.

25. Ibid.

26. Ibid.

27. Ibid., 61–62.

28. Ibid., 68.

29. Ibid., 69.

30. Ibid., 68.
31. Ibid., 70
32. Ibid., 155.
33. "A Good Report," *British Medical Journal* 2 (April 26, 1975): 155.
34. "Towards a Reborn G.M.C.," *The Lancet* (April 19, 1975): 901.
35. "A Good Report." *British Medical Journal* 2 (April 26, 1975): 155.
36. *Annual Report of the General Medical Council* (1975), 2.
37. "Towards a Reborn G.M.C."
38. "Merrison Report and Overseas Doctors," *British Medical Journal* 4 (December 6, 1975): 579–80.
39. "Merrison Report and Asian Doctors," *British Medical Journal* 2 (May 3, 1975): 277.
40. "G.M.C. and Indian Doctors," *British Medical Journal* 2 (June 7, 1975): 563.
41. "Overseas Doctors," *British Medical Journal* 3 (August 2, 1975): 310.
42. GMC and Overseas Doctors," *British Medical Journal* 4 (October 25, 1975): 228.

Conclusion

1. The legislation affected the British territory of Hong Kong and independent successor states of the empire: India, Malaysia, Singapore, South Africa and Australia.
2. "Registration of Overseas Doctors," *The Lancet* 317 (June 13, 1981): 1301.
3. "UK Sets Tougher Rules for Overseas Doctors," ibid. 346 (November 18, 1995): 1354.
4. "UK Immigration for Doctors (Natalie Jane MacDonald)," ibid. 344 (August 20, 1994): 548–49.
5. See also Stephanie Snow and Emma Jones, "Immigration and the National Health Service: Putting History to the Forefront," *History and Policy* (March 2011): 7, http://www.historyandpolicy.org/policy-papers/papers/immigration-and-the-national-health-service-putting-history-to-the-forefron.
6. "Editorial: Overseas Doctors and the UK's National Health Service," *The Lancet* 370 (July 21, 2007): 194.

Bibliography

Primary Sources

National Archives

Cabinet Office (CAB) 75/12/52
Privy Council (PC) 8/457, 8/1078, 8/1112, 8/1115, 8/1125, 8/1158, 8/1294, 8/1364, 8/1394, 8/1395
Privy Office (PC) 8/1395.
Ministry of National Service 1/814; 833.
Ministry of Health (MH) 76/334; 149/1003, 1004, 1076, 1827, 1828, 1829, 1833, 1834; 153/466, 548, 700, 709, 770 773.

Royal College of Physicians

Minutes of the Comitia

Government Reports

Report of the Committee to Consider the Future Numbers of Practitioners and the Appropriate In
Take of Medical Students (London: Her Majesty's Stationary Office, 1957)
Report of the Joint Working Party on the Medical Staffing Structure in the Hospital Service
(London: Her Majesty's Stationary Office, 1961).
Report of the Committee of Inquiry into the Regulation of the Medical Profession (London:
Her Majesty's Stationary Office, 1974–75).
Royal Commission Appointed to Look into the Medical Acts (29, 1882)
Royal Commission on Medical Education, 1965–68 (London: Her Majesty's Stationary Office, 1968)
Special Report of the Select Committee on Medical Amendment Act (XII, 1878–79)

Published Sources

General Medical Council on Education and Registration (GMC)

Annual Report of the GMC for 1971–80 (1972–81)
Interim Report of the Special Committee on the Registration of Overseas Doctors (February 1972)
Memorandum by the GMC on the Registration Fees (1966)
Memorandum on the Registration of Commonwealth and Foreign Doctors (October 1967)
Minutes of the GMC (1858–1980)

Secondary Sources

Abel-Smith, Brian, and Kathleen Gales. *British Doctors at Home and Abroad.* Welwyn, UK: Published for the Social Administration Research Trust by Codicote Press, 1964.

Abugideri, Hibba. *Gender and the Making of Modern Medicine in Colonial Egypt.* Farnham, Surrey, UK: Ashgate, 2010.

Arnold, David. *The New Cambridge History of India.* Vol. 3, *Science, Technology and Medicine in Colonial India.* Cambridge: Cambridge University Press, 2000.

Baldwin, M. Page. "Subject to Empire: Married Women and the British Nationality and Status of Aliens Act." *Journal of British Studies* 40 (October 2001): 522–56.

Bartrip, Peter. *Themselves Writ Large: The British Medical Association, 1832–1966.* London: BMJ Publishing Group, 1996.

Beck, Boyde. "Imperialism and Professionalization: Dominion Registration and Canadian Physicians during the Boer War." *HSTC Bulletin: Journal of the History of Canadian Science, Technology and Medicine/HTSC Bulletin: Revue d'historie des science, des techniques et de la medicine au Canada* 8, no. 1 (26) (1984): 3–19.

Bell, Heather. *Frontiers of Medicine in the Anglo-Egyptian Sudan, 1899–1940.* Oxford: Clarendon Press, 1999.

Bonner, Thomas. *To the Ends of the Earth: Women's Search for Education in Medicine.* Cambridge, MA: Harvard University, 1992.

———. *Becoming a Physician: Medical Education in Britain, France, Germany and the United States.* Oxford: Oxford University Press, 1995.

Boog, William N. "Four Monopolies and the Surgeons of London and Edinburgh." *Journal of the History of Medicine* 25, no. 3 (July 1970): 311–22.

Bowers, John. *Medical Education in Japan.* New York: Harper & Row, 1965.

———. *When the Twain Meet: The Rise of Western Medicine in Japan.* Baltimore: Johns Hopkins University Press, 1980.

Bradley, James, Ann Crowther, and Marguerite Dupree. "Mobility and Selection in Scottish University Medical Education, 1858–1886." *Medical History* 40 (1996): 1–24.

Brand, Jeanne. *Doctors and the State: The British Medical Profession and Government Growth, 1870–1912.* Baltimore: Johns Hopkins University, 1965.

Brockliss, Laurence. "The Professions and National Identity." In *A Union of Multiple Identities: The British Isles, 1750–1850,* edited by Laurence Brockliss and David Eastwood, 9–28. Manchester, UK: Manchester University Press, 1997.

Burton, Antoinette. *Burdens of History: British Feminists, Indian Women, and Imperial Culture.* Chapel Hill: University of North Carolina Press, 1994.

———. "Contesting the Zenana: The Mission to Make 'Lady Doctors for India,' 1874–1885." *Journal of British Studies* 35 (July 1996): 368–97.

Cantlie, Sir Neil. *A History of the Army Medical Department.* Vol. 2. Edinburgh: Churchill Livingstone, 1974.

Collins, Kenneth. *Go and Learn: The International Story of Jews and Medicine in Scotland.* Aberdeen: Aberdeen University Press, 1988.

Crossman, Richard. *The Diaries of a Cabinet Minister.* Vol. 3, *Secretary of State for Social Service, 1968–1970.* London: Hamish Hamilton and Jonathan Cape, 1977.

Crozier, Anna. *Practicing Colonial Medicine: The Colonial Medical Service in East Africa.* London: I. B. Tauris, 2007.

De Barros, Juanita. "'Spreading Sanitary Enlightenment': Race, Identity, and the Emergence of a Creole Medical Profession in British Guiana." *Journal of British Studies* 42, no. 2 (2003): 488–96.

Decker, Karola. "Overseas doctors: past and present." In *Racism in Medicine.* Edited by Naaz Coker. 23–53. London: King's Fund, 2001.

———. "Divisions and Diversity: The Complexities of Medical Refuge in Britain, 1933–1948." *Bulletin of the History of Medicine* 77 (2003): 850–73.

Del Felice, Renzo. *The Jews in Fascist Italy.* New York: Enigma Books, 2001.

Digby, Anne. "'A Medical El Dorado'? Colonial Medical Incomes and Practice at the Cape." *Social History of Medicine* 8, no. 3 (1995): 453–79.

———. *The Evolution of British General Practice.* Oxford: Oxford University Press, 1999.

Digby, Anne, and Nick Bosanquet. "Doctors and Patients in an Era of National Health Insurance and Private Practice, 1918–1938." *Economic History Review* 41, no. 1 (1988): 74–94.

Durbach, Nadia. *Bodily Matters: The Anti-vaccination Movement in England, 1853–1907.* Durham, NC: Duke University Press, 2005.

Efron, John M. Efron. *Medicine and the German Jews: A History.* New Haven, CT: Yale University Press, 2001.

Ellis, Jack D. *The Physician-Legislator of France: Medicine and Politics in the Early Third Republic, 1870–1914.* Cambridge: Cambridge University Press, 1990).

Elton, Mary Ann. "Medicine." In *Careers of Professional Women,* edited by Rosalie Silverstone and Audrey Ward, 99–134. London: Croon Helm, 1980.

Endelman, Todd M. *The Jews of Britain, 1656 to 2000.* Berkeley: University of California Press, 2002.

Fette, Julie. *Exclusions Practicing Prejudice in French Law and Medicine, 1920–1945.* Ithaca, NY: Cornell University Press, 2012.

Fleetwood, John F. *The History of Medicine in Ireland.* Dublin: Skelling Press, 1983.

Flinn, M. W. "Medical Services under the New Poor Law." In *The New Poor Law in the Nineteenth Century,* edited by Derek Fraser. London: Macmillan, 1976.

Gale, T. S. "Official Medical Policy in British West Africa, 1870–1930." PhD diss., University of London, 1973.

Hall, Catherine. *Civilising Subjects: Metropole and Colony in the English Imagination, 1830–1867.* Chicago: University of Chicago Press, 2002.

Hall, Catherine, and Sonya Rose, eds. *At Home with Empire: Metropolitan Culture and the Imperial World.* Cambridge: Cambridge University Press, 2006.

Hamilton, David. *The Healers: A History of Medicine in Scotland.* Edinburgh: Canongate, 1981.

Hamowy, Ronald. *Canadian Medicine: A Study in Restricted Entry.* Vancouver: Fraser Institute, 1984.

Harrison, Mark. *Public Heath in British India: Anglo-Indian Preventive Medicine, 1859–1914.* Cambridge: Cambridge University Press, 1994.

———. *Medicine and Victory: British Military Medicine in the Second World War.* Oxford: Oxford University Press, 2004.

———. *The Medical War: British Military Medicine and the First World War.* Oxford: Oxford University Press, 2010.

Haynes, Douglas M. "Social Status and Imperial Service: Tropical Medicine and the British Medical Profession in the Nineteenth Century." In *Warm Climates and Western Medicine: the Emergence of Tropical Medicine, 1500–1900,* edited by David Arnold. Amsterdam: Rodopi, 1996.

———. *Imperial Medicine: Patrick Manson and the Conquest of Tropical Disease.* Philadelphia: University of Pennsylvania Press, 2001.

———. "Victorian Imperialism in the Making of the British Medical Profession: An Argument." In *Decentering Empire: Britain, India and the Transcolonial World,* edited by Durba Ghosh and Dane Kennedy, 130–56. Hyderabad, India: Orient Longman, 2006.

———. "The Persistence of Privilege: British Medical Qualifications and the Practice of Medicine in the Empire." In *Beyond Sovereignty: Britain, Empire and Transnationalism, c. 1880–1950,* edited by Kevin Grant, Philippa Levine, and Frank Trentmann. Houndsmills, Basingstoke, UK: Palgrave, 2007.

Hull, Andrew, and Sanjoy Bhattacharya. "Health Service Sepoys? A Review of the Role of South Asians in the United Kingdom, c. 1944–1980." History of Science Working Papers Series, 1 (Department of History of Science, IMF-CSIC, Barcelona, Spain, 2004).

Jeffery, Roger. "Recognizing India's Doctors: The Institutionalization of Medical Dependency, 1918–1939." *Modern Asian Studies* 13, no. 2 (April 1979): 301–26.

Jones, Emma L., and Stephanie J. Snow. *"Against the Odds": Black and Minority Ethnic Clinicians and Manchester, 1948–2009.* Manchester, UK: Manchester NHS Primary Care Trust, 2010.

Jones, Greta. "The Rockefeller Foundation and Medical Education in Ireland in the 1920s." *Irish Historical Studies* 30, no. 120 (November 1997): 564–80.

———. "'Strike out Boldly for the Prizes that are Available to You': Medical Emigration from Ireland, 1870–1905." *Medical History* 54, no. 1 (January 2010): 55–74.

Karatani, Rieko. *Defining British Citizenship: Empire, Commonwealth and Modern Britain.* London: Frank Cass, 2003.

Kehoe, S. Karly. "Accessing Empire: Irish Surgeons and the Royal Navy, 1840–1880." *Social History of Medicine* 26, no. 2 (September 2013): 202–24.

Kumar, Anil. *Medicine and the Raj: British Medical Policy in India, 1835–1911.* New Delhi: Sage, 1998.

Kyriakides, Christopher, and Satnam Virdee. "Migrant Labour. Racism and the British National Health Service." *Ethnicity and Health* 8, no. 4 (November 2003): 283–305.

Layton-Henry, Zig. "Immigration and the Heath Government." In *The Heath Government*, edited by Stuart Ball and Anthony Seldon, 215–34. Harlow, UK: Addison Wesley Longman Group, 1996.

Levine, Philippa. *Prostitution, Race & Politics: Policing Venereal Disease in the British Empire.* London: Routledge, 2003.

Lloyd, Christopher, and Jack Coulter. *Medicine and the Navy, 1815–1900.* Vol. 4. London: E & S Livingstone, 1963.

LoGerfo, James. "Sir William Dolben and 'The Cause of Humanity': The Passage of the Slave Trade Regulation Act of 1788." *Eighteenth Century Studies* 6, no. 4 (Summer 1973): 431–52.

London, Louise. *Whitehall and the Jews: British Immigration Policy, Jewish Refugees and the Holocaust.* Cambridge: Cambridge University Press, 2000.

MacDermot, H .E. *Sir Thomas Roddick: His Work in Medicine and Public Life.* Toronto: Macmillan, 1938.

Manderson, Lenore. *Sickness and the State: Health and Illness in Colonial Malaya, 1870–1940.* Cambridge: Cambridge University Press, 1996.

Ollivier, Maurice, ed. *The Colonial and Imperial Conferences, 1887–1939.* Pt. 2. Vol. 3. Ottawa: Edmond Cloutier, 1954.

Peterson, M. Jeanne. *The Medical Profession in Mid-Victorian London.* Berkeley: University of California Press, 1978.

Patton Jr., Adell. *Physicians, Colonial Racism, and Diaspora in West Africa.* Gainesville: University of Florida Press, 1997.

Paul, Kathleen. *Whitewashing Britain: Race and Citizenship in the Postwar Era.* Ithaca, NY: Cornell University Press, 1997.

Pensabene, T. S. *The Rise of the Medical Practitioner in Victoria.* Canberra: Australian National University, 1980.

Porter, Dorothy. "Stratification and Its Discontents: Professionalisation and Conflict in British Public Health Services, 1848–1914." In *A History of Education in Public Health*, edited by Elizabeth Fee and Roy Acheson. Oxford: Oxford University Press, 1991.

———. *Health, Civilization and the State: A History of Public Health from Ancient to Modern Times.* London: Routledge, 1999.

Pyke-Lees, Walter. *Centenary of the General Medical Council, 1858–1958: The History and Present Work of the Council.* London: GMC, 1959.

Richardson, Ruth. *Death, Dissection and the Destitute.* London: Routledge, 1987.

Roberts, M. J. D. "The Politics of Professionalization: MPs, Medical Men, and the 1858 Medical Act." *Medical History* 53 (2009): 37–56.

Roberts, Shirley. *Sophia Jex-Blake: A Woman Pioneer in Nineteenth Century Medical Reform.* London: Routledge, 1993.

Seale, John. "Medical Emigration rom Britain, 1930–1961." *British Medical Journal* 17 (March 1962): 782–86.

Sen Gupta, P. C. "Soorjo Coomar Goodeve Chuckerbutty: The First Indian Contributors to Modern Medical Science." *Medical History* 14 (1970): 183–90.

Sheridan, Richard B. *Doctors and Slaves: A Medical and Demographic History of Slavery in the British West Indies, 1680–1834.* Cambridge: Cambridge University Press, 1985.

Sinha, Mrinalini. *Colonial Masculinity: 'The Manly Englishmen' and the 'Effeminate Bengali' in the Late Nineteenth Century.* Manchester, UK: Manchester University Press, 1995.

Snow, Stephanie, and Emma Jones. "Immigration and the National Health Service: Putting History to the Forefront." *History and Policy* (March 2011). http://www.historyandpolicy.org/policy-papers/papers/immigration-and-the-national-health-service-putting-history-to-the-forefron).

Stacey, Margaret. *Regulating British Medicine: The General Medical Council.* Chichester, UK: John Wiley & Sons, 1992.

Swinfen, D. B. *Imperial Control of Colonial Legislation, 1813–1865: A Study of British Policy towards Colonial Legislative Powers.* Oxford: Clarendon Press, 1970.

Van Heyningen, E. B. "Agents of Empire: The Medical Profession in Cape Colony, 1880–1910." *Medical History* 33 (October 1989): 450–53.

Waddington, Ivan. *The Medical Profession in the Industrial Revolution.* Dublin: Gill and Macmillan, 1986.

Warner, John Harley. *The Therapeutic Perspective: Medical Practice, Knowledge, Identity in America, 1820–1885.* Cambridge, MA: Harvard University Press, 1986.

Weaver, John. "'A Glut on the Market': Medical Practice Laws and Treatment of Refugee Doctors in Australia and New Zealand, 1933–1942." Unpublished essay.

Weindling, Paul. "Medical Refugees and the Modernization of British Medicine, 1930–1960." *Social History of Medicine* 27, no. 33 (2009): 489–511.

Weisz, George. *Divide and Conquer: A Comparative History of Medical Specialization.* Oxford: Oxford University Press, 2006.

Widdess, J. D. H. *The Royal College of Surgeons in Ireland.* Dublin: Royal College of Surgeons in Ireland, 1984.

Index

An italicized page number indicates a table.

CPSIA information can be obtained
at www.ICGtesting.com
Printed in the USA
LVHW091911231220
675003LV00005B/107

9 781580 465816